Biosimilars Development Strategies

After 18 years since the first biosimilar was approved, a lot has changed, from the regulatory guidelines to the stakeholder perceptions about the safety and efficacy of biosimilars. However, the development costs remain high, preventing faster entry into markets with more than 200 choices. Analyzing the regulatory filings of all approved biosimilars in the US and EU, a deep analysis of the scientific principles and continuous challenges to the regulatory authorities have made it possible to plan the development on a fast track. This book teaches how to cut the current time and cost by more than 70%, based on the author's hands-on experience.

Features:

- Describes the emergence of biosimilars since the first publication of the recombinant engineering patent, as well as a listing of all approved recombinant products, their patent expiry, and their adoption across the globe.
- Provides a better understanding of the safety and efficacy of approved biosimilars.
- Global approval requires accommodating guidelines and detailed planning to avoid redundancy as well as high costs. The basic expectations of the agencies are presented here.
- Presents a detailed analysis of all EU- and FDA-approved products with a comparative analysis.
- Renowned author and entrepreneur in the field of drug discovery and production.

Biosimilars
Development Strategies
Fast to Market Approaches

Sarfaraz K. Niazi
Adjunct Professor at the University of Illinois

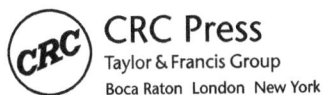

CRC Press
Taylor & Francis Group
Boca Raton London New York

CRC Press is an imprint of the
Taylor & Francis Group, an **informa** business

Cover illustration: Shutterstock—image number 369119591

First edition published in 2025
by CRC Press
2385 Executive Center Drive, Suite 320, Boca Raton, FL 33431

and by CRC Press
4 Park Square, Milton Park, Abingdon, Oxon, OX14 4RN

© 2025 Sarfaraz K. Niazi

CRC Press is an imprint of Taylor & Francis Group, LLC

ISBN: 9781032517018 (hbk)
ISBN: 9781032519586 (pbk)
ISBN: 9781003404637 (ebk)

DOI: 10.1201/9781003404637

Typeset in Times
by codeMantra

Contents

Preface

Biosimilars have come to the age of maturity with almost two decades behind them, yet unlike generic drugs, their scope is way behind what was expected when they were introduced. Less than 5% of available choices of biological drugs are currently available as biosimilars, entirely due to the higher cost and time it takes to develop biosimilars. This book is a practical guide to newcomers, as well as experienced developers, on optimizing their resources and understanding that it takes longer because of the amount of money that needs to be spent. So, taking a roundabout approach reduces the development cost and the time will follow—an extraordinary modeling approach.

Biosimilars are copies of biological products with no clinically meaningful difference from their reference product. Still, the lack of understanding about biological product safety has complicated their development cycle, which is the goal of this book to resolve.

Chapter 1: All About Biosimilars. It includes a list of 131 most essential summary articles on biosimilars.

Chapter 2: Product Type and Selection Strategies. Here, the developers will be educated about the choices available and provided metrics for selecting.

Chapter 3: Development Master Plan. A written signed-off plan is the best approach to start a project that will prove most efficient—unfortunately, this is one of the most neglected considerations by many.

Chapter 4: Optimization of Cost of Goods. Remember that in the end, you should be able to sell it at a 90% discount yet keep a 90% margin to succeed. This chapter teaches how to ensure both targets.

Chapter 5: Strategic Understanding of Biosimilar's Future. While the immediate interest is to bring more than 100 available choices to the market, future products, such as drug–antibody conjugates and likely other biological products added to the category of biosimilars, should be kept in mind.

Chapter 6: Repurposing Biosimilars. While developing a new biological drug remains a multibillion-dollar and a decade, an excellent opportunity for the newcomers is to find newer indications of the approved molecules. Unlike most think, this can be made into a very inexpensive exercise if planned correctly.

I have authored several books on the topic of biosimilars, as well as many papers; a bibliography at the end of the Preface should provide additional reference to expand this Preface.

I wish to thank many who have worked with me for decades in creating new biosimilars and other biotechnology products, and several continue to work with me. The attention I get from Sarah Yim and Janet Woodcock of the FDA is exemplary in ensuring that while the goal of the FDA is to ensure safety and efficacy, creativity at the FDA continues to optimize the cost of reaching that goal. Thanks to Sarah and Janet.

Sarfaraz K. Niazi,
Deerfield, Illinois

Author

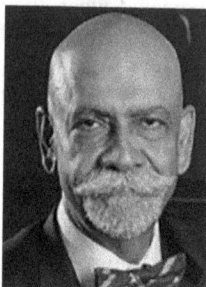

Sarfaraz K Niazi, Ph.D. is an adjunct professor at the University of Illinois. He has authored 60+ major books, 100+ research papers, and 100+ patents, mainly in bioprocessing. He has hands-on experience establishing biopharmaceutical projects, from concept to market, including setting up the first biosimilar company in the US and leading to several FDA approvals. He serves as an advisor to several regulatory agencies, including the FDA.

1 All About Biosimilars

1.1 INTRODUCTION

New drug development costs now run into billions of dollars, leading to their high price for at least 5 years for a new chemical and 12 years for a new biological drug. In addition, the stringent regulatory guidelines have raised the cost of a new biological drug approval to hundreds of millions USD, resulting in the high price of these products (Table 1.1) to amortize the investment over the 12 years of exclusivity for biological drugs.

TABLE 1.1
Most Expensive Treatment Costs of Therapeutic Proteins

Drug	Active	Indication	Cost, USD
Actemra	Tocilizumab	Rheumatoid arthritis and cytokine release syndrome	6,000–9,000/month
Actimmune	Interferon gamma-1b	Chronic granulomatous disease and severe, malignant osteopetrosis	157,000/year
Blenrep	Belantamab mafodotin	Multiple myeloma	400,000/year
Blincyto	Blinatumomab	Acute lymphoblastic leukemia (ALL)	178,000/trt
Brineura	Cerliponase alfa	Late infantile neuronal ceroid lipofuscinosis type 2 (CLN2)	350,000/year
Ceredase	Alglucerase	Gaucher disease	200,000–300,000/year
Cerezyme	Imiglucerase	Gaucher disease	350,000/year
Darzalex	Daratumumab	Multiple myeloma	150,000–170,000/year
Elaprase	Idursulfase	Hunter syndrome (MPS II)	375,000/year
Erwinaze	Asparaginase erwinia chrysanthemi	Acute lymphoblastic leukemia (ALL)	14,000–28,000 per vial.
Hemlibra	Emicizumab	Prevention of bleeding episodes in hemophilia A with factor VIII inhibitors	482,000/year
Ilaris	Canakinumab	Cryopyrin-associated periodic syndromes (CAPS) and systemic juvenile idiopathic arthritis	200,000–300,000/year
Imfinzi	Durvalumab	Certain types of cancer, including lung cancer	150,000–170,000/year

(Continued)

DOI: 10.1201/9781003404637-1

TABLE 1.1 (Continued)
Most Expensive Treatment Costs of Therapeutic Proteins

Drug	Active	Indication	Cost, USD
Keytruda	Pembrolizumab	Various types of cancer, including melanoma and lung cancer	150,000–170,000/year
Kyprolis	Carfilzomib	Multiple myeloma	180,000–200,000/year
Monjuvi	Tafasitamab	Diffuse large B- cell lymphoma	$160,000/year
Naglazyme	Galsulfase	Mucopolysaccharidosis VI (MPS VI)	375,000/year
Ocrevus	Ocrelizumab	Multiple sclerosis	65,000/year
Opdivo	Nivolumab	Various types of cancer, including melanoma and lung cancer	150,000–170,000/year
Opdivo plus	Nivolumab + Ipilimumab	Certain types of cancer, including melanoma and lung cancer	250,000–270,000/year
Padcev	Enfortumab vedotin	Urothelial cancer	16,000/ month
Pulmozyme	Dornase alfa	Cystic fibrosis	311,000/year
Remicade	Infliximab	Rheumatoid arthritis, Crohn's disease, and other autoimmune conditions	30,000–40,000/year
Soliris	Eculizumab	Paroxysmal nocturnal hemoglobinuria (PNH) and atypical hemolytic uremic syndrome (ahus)	500,000–700,000/year
Stelara	Ustekinumab	Psoriasis, psoriatic arthritis, and Crohn's disease	30,000–40,000/year
Strensiq	Asfotase alfa	Hypophosphatasia	300,000/year
Synagis	Palivizumab	Prevention of respiratory syncytial virus (RSV) in infants	9,000–15,000 per month during RSV season.
Takhzyro	Lanadelumab	Hereditary angioedema	488,000/year
Tecentriq	Atezolizumab	Certain types of cancer, including bladder cancer	150,000–170,000/year
Ultomiris	Ravulizumab	Paroxysmal nocturnal hemoglobinuria (PNH) and atypical hemolytic uremic syndrome (ahus)	498,000/year
Vimizim	Elosulfase alfa	Morquio A syndrome	375,000/year
Xolair	Omalizumab	Severe asthma and chronic idiopathic urticaria	32,500/year
Yervoy	Ipilimumab	Certain types of cancer, including melanoma	150,000–170,000/year

1.2 APPROVALS

As the patents expire on a new biological drug, its biosimilars enter the market, a history that is remarkable in its span but also shaky in the extent to which the biosimilars have entered the market. A severe deficiency in the biosimilar landscape is the dearth of molecules entering the market; so far, only 14 molecules are available in the USA and 14 in the EU, while many remarkable choices await entry (Tables 1.2–1.4)

TABLE 1.2
Lists the 41 FDA Approvals of Biosimilars; There were no Rejections or Withdrawals Reported (1)

No	Biosimilar Name	Approval Date	Reference Product
1.	Tyruko (natalizumab-stn)	August 2023	Tysabri (natalizumab)
2.	Yuflyma (adalimumab-aaty)	May 2023	Humira (adalimumab)
3.	Idacio (adalimumab-aacf)	December 2022	Humira (adalimumab)
4.	Vegzelma (bevacizumab-adcd)	September 2022	Avastin (bevacizumab)
5.	Stimufend (pegfilgrastim-fpgk)	September 2022	Neulasta (pegfilgrastim)
6.	Cimerli (ranibizumab-eqrn)	August 2022	Lucentis (ranibizumab)
7.	Fylnetra (pegfilgrastim-pbbk)	May 2022	Neulasta (pegfilgrastim)
8.	Alymsys (bevacizumab-maly)	April 2022	Avastin (bevacizumab)
9.	Releuko (filgrastim-ayow)	February 2022	Neupogen (filgrastim)
10.	Yusimry (adalimumab-aqvh)	December 2021	Humira (adalimumab)
11.	Rezvoglar (insulin glargine-aglr)	December 2021	Lantus (insulin glargine)
12.	Byooviz (ranibizumab-nuna)	September 2021	Lucentis (ranibizumab)
13.	Semglee (Insulin glargine-yfgn)	July 2021	Lantus (Insulin glargine)
14.	Riabni (rituximab-arrx)	December 2020	Rituxan (rituximab)
15.	Hulio (adalimumab-fkjp)	July 2020	Humira (adalimumab)
16.	Nyvepria (pegfilgrastim-apgf)	June 2020	Neulasta (pegfilgrastim)
17.	Avsola (infliximab-axxq)	December 2019	Remicade (infliximab)
18.	Abrilada (adalimumab-afzb)	November 2019	Humira (adalimumab)
19.	Ziextenzo (pegfilgrastim-bmez)	November 2019	Neulasta (pegfilgrastim)
20.	Hadlima (adalimumab-bwwd)	July 2019	Humira (adalimumab)
21.	Ruxience (rituximab-pvvr)	July 2019	Rituxan (rituximab)
22.	Zirabev (bevacizumab-bvzr)	June 2019	Avastin (bevacizumab)
23.	Kanjinti (trastuzumab-anns)	June 2019	Herceptin (trastuzumab)
24.	Eticovo (etanercept-ykro)	April 2019	Enbrel (etanercept)
25.	Trazimera (trastuzumab-qyyp)	March 2019	Herceptin (trastuzumab)
26.	Ontruzant (trastuzumab-dttb)	January 2019	Herceptin (trastuzumab)
27.	Herzuma (trastuzumab-pkrb)	December 2018	Herceptin (trastuzumab)
28.	Truxima (rituximab-abbs)	November 2018	Rituxan (rituximab)
29.	Udenyca (pegfilgrastim-cbqv)	November 2018	Neulasta (pegfilgrastim)
30.	Hyrimoz (adalimumab-adaz)	October 2018	Humira (adalimumab)
31.	Nivestym (filgrastim-aafi)	July 2018	Neupogen (filgrastim)

(Continued)

TABLE 1.2 *(Continued)*

Lists the 41 FDA Approvals of Biosimilars; There were no Rejections or Withdrawals Reported (1)

No	Biosimilar Name	Approval Date	Reference Product
32.	Fulphila (pegfilgrastim-jmdb)	June 2018	Neluasta (pegfilgrastim)
33.	Retacrit (epoetin alfa-epbx)	May 2018	Epogen (epoetin-alfa)
34.	i. Ixifi (infliximab-qbtx)	December 2017	Remicade (infliximab)
35.	Ogivri (trastuzumab-dkst)	December 2017	Herceptin (trastuzumab)
36.	ii. Mvasi (Bevacizumab-awwb)	September 2017	Avastin (bevacizumab)
37.	Cyltezo (Adalimumab-adbm)	August 2017	Humira (adalimumab)
38.	Renflexis (Infliximab-abda)	May 2017	Remicade (infliximab)
39.	Amjevita (Adalimumab-atto)	September 2016	Humira (adalimumab)
40.	Erelzi (Etanercept-szzs)	August 2016	Enbrel (etanercept)
41.	Inflectra (Infliximab-dyyb)	April 2016	Remicade (infliximab)
42.	Zarxio (Filgrastim-sndz)	March 2015	Neupogen (filgrastim)

TABLE 1.3

Biosimilars Approved, Rejected, and Withdrawn in the EU [https://www.gabionline.net/biosimilars/general/biosimilars-approved-in-europe]

No.	Product Name	Active Substance	Authorization Date
1.	Vegzelma	Bevacizumab	22 Mar 2023
2.	Sondelbay	Teriparatide	16 Jun 2022
3.	Stimufend	Pegfilgrastim	12 Mar 2022
4.	Hukyndra	Adalimumab	15 Nov 2021
5.	Libmyris	Adalimumab	12 Nov 2021
6.	Byooviz	Ranibizumab	18 Aug 2021
7.	Abevmy	Bevacizumab	21 Apr 2021
8.	Alymsys	Bevacizumab	26 Mar 2021
9.	Oyavas	Bevacizumab	26 Mar 2021
10.	Yuflyma	Adalimumab	11 Feb 2021
11.	Kirsty (previously Kixelle)	Insulin aspart	5 February 2021
12.	Onbevzi	Bevacizumab	11 Jan 2021
13.	Nyvepria	Pegfilgrastim	18 Nov 2020
14.	Livogiva	Teriparatide	27 Aug 2020
15.	Aybintio	Bevacizumab	19 Aug 2020
16.	Zercepac	Trastuzumab	27 Jul 2020
17.	Insulin aspart Sanofi	Insulin aspart	25 Jun 2020
18.	Nepexto	Etanercept	25 May 2020
19.	Ruxience	Rituximab	1 Apr 2020
20.	Amsparity	Adalimumab	13 Feb 2020
21.	Cegfila	Pegfilgrastim	19 Dec 2019
22.	Grasustek	Pegfilgrastim	20 Jun 2019

(Continued)

TABLE 1.3 (*Continued*)
Biosimilars Approved, Rejected, and Withdrawn in the EU [https://www.gabionline.net/biosimilars/general/biosimilars-approved-in-europe]

No.	Product Name	Active Substance	Authorization Date
23.	Idacio	Adalimumab	2 Apr 2019
24.	Zirabev	Bevacizumab	14 Feb 2019
25.	Ogivri	Trastuzumab	12 Dec 2018
26.	Ziextenzo	Pegfilgrastim	22 Nov 2018
27.	Fulphila	Pegfilgrastim	20 Nov 2018
28.	Pelmeg	Pegfilgrastim	20 Nov 2018
29.	Pelgraz	Pegfilgrastim	21 Sep 2018
30.	Hulio	Adalimumab	17 Sep 2018
31.	Hefiya	Adalimumab	26 Jul 2018
32.	Hyrimoz	Adalimumab	26 Jul 2018
33.	Trazimera	Trastuzumab	26 Jul 2018
34.	Zessly	Infliximab	18 May 2018
35.	Kanjinti	Trastuzumab	16 May 2018
36.	Semglee	Insulin glargine	28 Mar 2018
37.	Herzuma	Trastuzumab	8 Feb 2018
38.	Mvasi	Bevacizumab	15 Jan 2018
39.	Ontruzant	Trastuzumab	15 Nov 2017
40.	Imraldi	Adalimumab	24 Aug 2017
41.	Insulin lispro Sanofi	Insulin lispro	18 Jul 2017
42.	Blitzima	Rituximab	13 Jul 2017
43.	Erelzi	Etanercept	23 Jun 2017
44.	Rixathon	Rituximab	15 Jun 2017
45.	Riximyo	Rituximab	15 Jun 2017
46.	Enoxaparin BECAT	Enoxaparin sodium	24 Mar 2017
47.	Amgevita	Adalimumab	21 Mar 2017
48.	Truxima	Rituximab	17 Feb 2017
49.	Movymia	Teriparatide	11 Jan 2017
50.	Terrosa	Teriparatide	4 Jan 2017
51.	Inhixa	Enoxaparin sodium	15 Sep 2016
52.	Flixabi	Infliximab	26 May 2016
53.	Benepali	Etanercept	13 Jan 2016
54.	Accofil	Filgrastim	17 Sep 2014
55.	Abasaglar	Insulin glargine	9 Sep 2014
56.	Bemfola	Follitropin alfa	26 Mar 2014
57.	Grastofil	Filgrastim	17 Oct 2013
58.	Ovaleap	Follitropin alfa	27 Sep 2013
59.	Inflectra	Infliximab	10 Sep 2013
60.	Remsima	Infliximab	10 Sep 2013
61.	Nivestim	Filgrastim	7 Jun 2010
62.	Filgrastim hexal	Filgrastim	6 Feb 2009
63.	Zarzio	Filgrastim	6 Feb 2009
64.	Ratiograstim	Filgrastim	15 Sep 2008

(*Continued*)

TABLE 1.3 (*Continued*)
Biosimilars Approved, Rejected, and Withdrawn in the EU [https://www.gabionline.net/biosimilars/general/biosimilars-approved-in-europe]

No.	Product Name	Active Substance	Authorization Date
65.	Tevagrastim	Filgrastim	15 Sep 2008
66.	Retacrit	Epoetin zeta	18 Dec 2007
67.	Silapo	Epoetin zeta	18 Dec 2007
68.	Binocrit	Epoetin alfa	28 Aug 2007
69.	Abseamed	Epoetin alfa	27 Aug 2007
70.	Epoetin alfa hexal	Epoetin alfa	27 Aug 2007
71.	Omnitrope	Somatropin	12 Apr 2006
	Refused or Withdrawn Biosimilars in Europe		
1.	Alpheon	Interferon alfa-2a	Refused 5 Sep 2006
2.	Biograstim	Filgrastim	15 Sep 2008; Withdrawn on 22 Dec 2016
3.	Cyltezo	Adalimumab	10 Nov 2017 Withdrawn on 15 Jan 2019
4.	Epostim	Epoetin alfa	Withdrawn 15 Mar 2011
5.	Equidacent	Bevacizumab	24 Sep 2020 Withdrawn on 23 Nov 2021
6.	Filgrastim ratiopharm	Filgrastim	15 Sep 2008; Withdrawn on 20 Apr 2011
7.	Halimatoz	Adalimumab	26 Jul 2018; Withdrawn on 29 Jan 2021
8.	Kromeya	Adalimumab	2 Apr 2019; Withdrawn on 17 Dec 2019
9.	Lextemy	Bevacizumab	CHMP positive opinion 25 Feb 2021; Withdrawn on 14 Dec 2021
10.	Lusduna	Insulin glargine	3 Jan 2017; Withdrawn on 29 Oct 2018
11.	Qutavina	Teriparatide	27 Aug 2020; Withdrawn on 18 Jan 2021
12.	Ritemvia	Rituximab	13 Jul 2017; Withdrawn on 16 Aug 2021
13.	Rituximab mabion	Rituximab	Withdrawn on 16 Mar 2020
14.	Rituzena	Rituximab	13 Jul 2017; Withdrawn on 10 Apr 2019
15.	Solumarv	Insulin human	Refused 11 Feb 2016
16.	Sondelbay	Teriparatide	Withdrawn on 19 Jun 2020
17.	Solymbic	Adalimumab	22 Mar 2017; Withdrawn on 5 Mar 2019
18.	Somatropin biopartners	Somatropin	9 Sep 2013; Withdrawn on 9 Nov 2017
19.	Thorinane	Enoxaparin sodium	14 Sep 2016; Withdrawn on 24 Oct 2019
20.	Udenyca	Pegfilgrastim	21 Sep 2018; Withdrawn on 15 Feb 2021
21.	Valtropin	Somatropin	24 Apr 2006; Withdrawn on 10 May 2012

1.3   FUTURE CANDIDATES

TABLE 1.4
Potential Biosimilar Candidates (https://www.drugpatentwatch.com)

Abatacept	Abciximab	Aflibercept	Alemtuzumab
Alirocumab	Atezolizumab	Avelumab	Basiliximab
Bedinvetman (V)	Belimumab	Benralizumab	Bevacizumab
Bezlotoxumab	Blinatumomab	Blood factors	Brentuximab vedotin

(Continued)

TABLE 1.4 *(Continued)*
Potential Biosimilar Candidates (https://www.drugpatentwatch.com)

Abatacept	Abciximab	Aflibercept	Alemtuzumab
Brodalumab	Brolucizumab	Burosumab	Canakinumab
Caplacizumab	Cemiplimab	Certolizumab pegol	Cetuximab
Crizanlizumab	Daclizumab	Daratumumab	Darbepoetin alfa
Denosumab	Dinutuximab	Dupilumab	Durvalumab
Eculizumab	Elotuzumab	Emapalumab	Emicizumab
Erenumab	Etanercept	Evolocumab	Follitropin alfa
Fremanezumab	Frunevetmab (V)	Galcanezumab	Gemtuzumab ozogamicin
Golimumab	Guselkumab	Ibalizumab	Idarucizumab
Inotuzumab ozogamicin	Insulin detemir	Insulin lispro	Interferons
Ipilimumab	Isatuximab	Ixekizumab	Lanadelumab
Lokivetab (V)	Mepolizumab	ogamulizumab	Moxetumomab pasudodox
Muromonab-CD3	Natalizumab	Necitumumab	Nivolumab
Obiltoxaximab	Obinutuzumab	Ocrelizumab	Ofatumumab
Olaratumab	Omalizumab	Palivizumab	Panitumumab
Pembrolizumab	Pertuzumab	Polatuzumab vedotin	Ramucirumab
Ranibizumab	Ravulizumab	Raxibacumab	Reslizumab
Rilonacept	Risankizumab	Romosozumab	Sacituzumab govitecan-hziy
Sarilumab	Secukinumab	Selumetinib	Siltuximab
Teprotumumab-trbw	Tildrakizumab	Tocilizumab	Urofollitropin

1.4   APPROVAL GUIDELINES

The first tranche of biosimilar approval guidelines treated biosimilars like new biological drugs for an abundance of caution, including extensive analytical comparisons, animal pharmacology and toxicology, clinical pharmacology, and clinical safety and efficacy studies. The only concession allowed is the extrapolation of indications. A comparative clinical efficacy testing in one indication would be sufficient to qualify for all indications allowed for the reference product. To further assure safety and efficacy, biosimilars must have the same dose, strength, route of administration, and mechanism of action; the formulations may differ. Also, the prescribing information must be the same, and guidelines are available on writing the prescribing information for biosimilars.

Over time, the agencies became more convinced of the safety of biosimilars in response to challenges made to the guidelines. It became well accepted that the animal testing of biosimilars is redundant since now even the new biological products may not be required to conduct such testing because the mechanism of action of biological drugs involves receptor binding that is often unavailable in animal species. The value of clinical efficacy testing has also come under criticism for scientific reasons since these studies cannot fail and, if used to overcome a lack of similarity in analytical or clinical pharmacology, create a higher safety risk possibility if these studies are considered for approval. An excellent example of progressive changes to guidelines comes from the Medicines and Healthcare products Regulatory Agency (MHRA). Last year, as the Brexit transition period ended, the MHRA published its first comprehensive guideline on May 14, 2022, that breaks from all other guidelines by providing clear judgment for not requiring animal and clinical efficacy studies.

Clinical pharmacology studies, including pharmacokinetic and pharmacodynamic (PD) comparisons, are part of the analytical methodologies, where we establish similarities in how the body sees the drug and vice versa. These should be enhanced and recommended for newer technologies and approaches to develop structural equivalence.

Other misconceptions include animal testing and clinical efficacy testing. At the end of 2022, the US government passed a new law, the FDA Modernization Act 2.0, removing the term "animal toxicology" and replacing it with "nonclinical" to remove all animal testing since animals do not have the receptors to respond to biological drugs. In addition, the MHRA recently announced that animal and clinical efficacy testing might be unnecessary. This will be the first requirement for any universal guideline to remove all animal testing; if used to justify the variability in analytical assessment, as commonly practiced, animal testing creates a risk of approval of unsafe biosimilars.

The limitations of efficacy testing in patients are well recognized by regulatory agencies. To overcome these concerns, the FDA's Division of Applied Regulatory Science (DARS) has recently published its recommendations to remove this testing for biosimilars based on comparing PD properties between a biosimilar candidate and its reference product. It is now labeled as clinical efficacy testing in healthy subjects. A PD biomarker is not required to be a surrogate endpoint or have an established relationship with clinical efficacy outcomes. Examples include the absolute neutrophil count area under the effect time curve as a more reliable endpoint than the clinical efficacy endpoint of the duration of severe neutropenia. DARS made these conclusions based on its investigations and clinical studies it has conducted to define the best practices for characterizing the PD biomarkers for various drug classes. These studies evaluated the use of human plasma proteomic and transcriptomic analysis to find novel biomarkers for the approval of biosimilars. More efforts are underway to remove patient testing of all biological drugs, including monoclonal antibodies that do not show PD markers.

The clinical efficacy trials have not revealed any clinically significant differences between a biosimilar and its reference product, according to a review of the published literature. Therefore, they have not led to any product withdrawals or recalls from the market. These data are available in the 96 European public assessment reports (EPAR) files from the European Medicines Agency EMA and 37 approval documents from the FDA. These regulatory submissions all passed their clinical efficacy assessment. In addition, the research published on the clinicaltrials.gov website substantiates that all 141 studies provided the findings complied with the required standards. The PubMed database also provides 435 randomized control clinical trials conducted between 2002 and 2022 which failed to detect a clinically significant difference.

The main reason to remove clinical efficacy testing is not cost avoidance; it is based on ethical concerns that arise from the universal belief that no unnecessary exposure to healthy subjects should be made as codified in the US 21 CFR 320.25(a)(13), the universal belief that "No unnecessary human testing should be performed." The hazardous concerns arise from the possibility of approving biosimilars based on clinical efficacy testing, overruling the mismatches in analytical and clinical pharmacology profiles.

The FDA now allows waiving efficacy testing in patients based on comparing PD properties between a biosimilar candidate and its reference product. It is now labeled as clinical efficacy testing in healthy subjects. A PD biomarker is not required to be a surrogate endpoint or have an established relationship with clinical efficacy outcomes. Examples include the absolute neutrophil count area under the effect time curve as a more reliable endpoint than the clinical efficacy endpoint of the duration of severe neutropenia. The PD biomarker identification can be made using large-scale proteomic approaches and other technologies where PD biomarkers are not readily available. The FDA has also confirmed that the PD biomarkers need not correlate with a clinical response to allow their use to support the claim of biosimilarity. A biosimilar development plan aims to demonstrate similarity to the reference product, not the focus of the reference product, where the safety and effectiveness are established independently. Therefore, the correlation between the PD biomarker and clinical outcomes, while beneficial, is not required.

If discrepancies exist between a proposed biosimilar and its reference product, Pharmacokinetic (PK) and PD similarity analysis may be more sensitive than clinical effectiveness endpoint (s) analysis to establish biosimilarity. The standards for surrogate biomarkers used to support the approval of novel drugs are fundamentally different from the standards for PD biomarkers meant to assist a demonstration of biosimilarity. This provides opportunities for biomarkers used as secondary and exploratory endpoints in new drug development programs to support biosimilar testing. In addition, many opportunities are available to identify new PD biomarkers or fill information gaps on existing biomarkers to facilitate using PD biomarker data in clinical pharmacology studies instead of comparative clinical efficacy studies.

1.5 WAIVERS

Possible examples of drugs that exhibit PD markers and thus are exempt from patient testing are presented in Table 1.5.

TABLE 1.5
Biosimilars with PD Markers Are Exempted from Clinical Efficacy Testing in Patients

Drug	Patent Expiry
Interferon beta-1b	2004
Parathyroid hormone	2004
Interferon alfa-2b	2004
Chorionic gonadotropin	2007
Interferon alfa-n3	2011
Etanercept	2012
Menotropins	2015
Urofollitropin	2015
Peginterferon alfa-2b	2015
Interferon beta-1a	2020
Insulin regular	2025
Insulin lispro	2014

For products that do not display PD biomarkers, such as monoclonal antibodies, other "omic" technologies like transcriptomics and metabolomics may offer a chance to find new, sensitive, and robust candidate biomarkers for further exploration as PD biomarkers. However, a more rational approach will be to take a step back in the testing cycle of biosimilars and examine if ex vivo testing can provide evidence of biosimilarity that is more sensitive and reliable in identifying any "clinically meaningful difference" in the language of the FDA guidelines.

Since the PD response is triggered by receptor binding, cell-based bioassays, or potency assays, such as ELISA, binding assays, competitive assays, cell signaling, ligand binding, proliferation, and proliferation suppression, should provide a good functional comparison of a biosimilar candidate with its reference product. Furthermore, functional tests for the mode of action, such as testing for apoptosis, complement-dependent cytotoxicity, antibody-dependent cellular phagocytosis, and antibody-dependent cellular cytotoxicity, are generally not required and can be added to provide a higher degree of confidence in safety and efficacy.

A collection of functional assays pertinent to a range of biological activities can be employed for a product having multiple biological activities. For instance, some proteins have a variety of functional domains that express enzymatic and receptor-binding functions. The metric for biological activity is potency. Analytical studies to evaluate these features are easily accessible when immunochemical properties are made part of the activity assigned to the product (for instance, antibodies or antibody-based products). The functional assays form more robust markers to establish efficacy comparisons than the testing in patients, without the necessity to demonstrate any PD response for mABs.

1.6　APPENDIX 1: TERMINOLOGY

The regulatory guidelines and standard scientific literature relating to biosimilars have adopted a specific vocabulary, as described in Table 1.6.[1]

TABLE 1.6

Terminology Related to Biosimilars

Biobetter	A biological product cannot claim to be a proposed biosimilar product if it has higher efficacy, lower dose requirement, fewer side effects, more convenient drug administration, or any other difference considered an improvement over the reference product. Such products are considered new biological products and are not accepted for evaluation by agencies under this guideline.
Comparability Testing	Comparability guidance such as ICH Q5E and ICH Q6B applies to a change in the manufacturing process of an approved product. The testing is conducted using the final approved biological product as the reference product. The testing is limited to critical-quality attributes that are well-known to the manufacturer. These guidelines may serve as overall guidance but do not apply to biosimilars development, any stage of development, including the final scale-up. However, the agencies' guidance may apply once the product has been approved. To avoid any confusion in referring to these guidelines, the current guideline uses the term "comparative testing" rather than "comparability testing."

(Continued)

TABLE 1.6 (*Continued*)
Terminology Related to Biosimilars

Product	When used without modifiers, it is intended to refer to the intermediates, drug substances, and drug products, as appropriate. The use of the term product is consistent with the use of the term in ICH Q5E. This should not be confused with the regulatory consideration of a drug or a biological product's approval pathway. A drug product can be approved as a drug or as a biological product. During the development process, a biological proposed is labeled by adding "proposed" to differentiate it from a proposed biosimilar that will be an authorized product.
High Similarity or Highly Similar	The similarity is a binomial attribute; a protocol for testing may fail or pass. If it fails, a close examination is conducted to determine the cause of failure, if any of the failed attributes have clinical significance. Often the terms "high similarity" or "highly similar" are used to indicate that there is residual uncertainty remaining that is clinically meaningful.
No clinically meaningful differences	A proposed biosimilar product is not identical to the reference product. There are differences with the reference product; if the differences do not affect safety or efficacy, we can claim no clinically meaningful difference.
No residual uncertainty	Every test must meet a pre-determined qualification; however, where the testing fails, it leaves uncertainty about the safety and efficacy as supported by the given test. When such delays are removed, we can call that a test left no residual uncertainty.
No one size fits all	Every testing of biosimilars is specific to the product type and requires highly individualized development protocols.
Fingerprint-like similarity	At the highest possible level, a similarity level is the only variance remaining in the analytical methodology variations. In most cases, reaching this level of similarity will significantly reduce the burden of additional testing.
Totality-of-the-evidence	The evidence of safety and clinical efficacy is accumulated through multiple studies, and when we combine all results, we can establish biosimilarity.
Stepwise	Testing is conducted in pre-defined steps, and only when the testing meets the criterion at one step that the testing can move to the next step; there is the significance of a higher value of any test, and a higher step does not resolve residual uncertainties of the lower steps.
Phase 1–3 studies	Phase studies, 1–3, are either stand-alone, 1 and 2, or placebo control, as in phase 3. None of these conditions apply to any testing of proposed biosimilar products; these terms are widely used by regulatory agencies and mostly by developers. The correct designations are nonclinical pharmacology, clinical pharmacology, or comparative efficacy studies
Joint Meeting	Regulators at both the European Medicines Agency (EMA) and the US Food and Drug Administration (FDA) support and foster increasingly globalized approaches to medicines development. Covering a broad range of relevant topics in medicines development, both agencies participate in multilateral fora such as the International Council on Harmonization (ICH), the International Coalition of Medicines Regulatory Authorities (ICMRA), and the World Health Organization (WHO) to address topics such as standards setting and policy convergence at the global level. On a smaller scale, the two agencies lead more than 30 technical working groups or "clusters" where members exchange perspectives and experiences on regulatory science topics. The cluster meetings are opportunities for regulatory experts to discuss amongst themselves challenges and difficult applications of regulatory

(Continued)

TABLE 1.6 (Continued)
Terminology Related to Biosimilars

Joint Meeting science and policy based on the priorities of the Agencies and are not intended to serve as a forum for advising sponsors. There are situations, however, in which a developer can benefit from scientific advice on a product development program from both agencies concurrently, and where convergent advice on the same or similar product-based scientific questions could benefit public health and facilitate patient access to needed therapies. To meet this need, EMA and FDA established a sponsor-initiated, product-specific exchange: the parallel scientific advice (PSA) program.

PSA provides a mechanism for EMA and FDA experts, upon request by the applicant, to concurrently advise sponsors on scientific issues during the development of new medicinal products (drugs, biologicals, vaccines, and advanced therapies). Importantly, as part of the process, the two agencies engage with each other to compare perspectives in advance of and during the actual interaction with the sponsor. This voluntary program was launched in 2005 with four goals: increase dialog between the two agencies and sponsors from the beginning of the lifecycle of a new product; provide a deeper understanding of the bases of regulatory decisions; optimize product development; and avoid unnecessary testing.

To initiate a PSA request, the applicant, herein referred to as "sponsor," emails a request to each agency. The request is expected to be brief and state the rationale for why the PSA would be beneficial, the proposed scientific questions to the agencies, and the desired goals for the meeting. If both agencies agree to accept the request, the sponsor can move forward with preparing a full meeting package according to EMA's Scientific Advice Working Party (SAWP) procedure schedule. A bilateral meeting between the EMA and the FDA takes place approximately 35 days after the EMA validates the meeting package. After the bilateral meeting, preliminary feedback from each agency is shared with the sponsor in writing. This could include preliminary responses to the sponsor's questions or requests for the sponsor to clarify or expand a concept or proposed pathway. At approximately 65 days after validation, a trilateral meeting with the sponsor, EMA, and FDA is held. Written advice from each agency to the sponsor follows this meeting, from EMA within 10 days and 30 days from FDA.

1.7 APPENDIX 2: THERAPEUTIC PROTEINS APPROVED BY THE FDA: POTENTIAL BIOSIMILAR CANDIDATES

Name	Accession No.	BLA / NDA	Brand Name	Type of Molecule	AA#	MW
Abatacept	DB01281	125118/S-240	Orencia	Fusion protein	357	39.45
Adalimumab	DB00051	125057/46	Humira	Monoclonal Antibody	665	72.72

(Continued)

Name	Accession No.	BLA / NDA	Brand Name	Type of Molecule	AA#	MW
Aducanumab	D10541	761178	Aduhelm	Monoclonal Antibody	667	72.95
Aflibercept	D09574	125387/S-061	Eylea	Fusion protein	431	48.46
Agalsidase Beta	DB00103	103979/ S-5309	Fabrazyme	Enzyme	398	45.35
Albiglutide	DB09043	125431/0	Tanzeum	Fusion protein	645	73.01
Aldesleukin	DB00041	103293/5114	Proleukin	Cytokine	133	15.46
Alefacept	DB00092	125036/142	Amevive	Fusion protein	707	79.93
Alemtuzumab	3A189DH42V	103948	Campath, Lemtrada	Monoclonal Antibody	666	73.03
Alglucerase	DB00088	NDA 20-057/S-034	Ceredase	Enzyme	497	55.60
Alirocumab	D10335	125559	Praluent	Monoclonal Antibody	667	72.99
Alpha-1-proteinase inhibitor	DB00058	125039	Aralast, Glassia, Prolastin, Prolastin-C, Respreeza, Zemaira	Inhibitors	225	29.07
Alteplase	DB00009	103172	Activase	Enzyme	527	59.04
Anakinra	DB00026	103950/ S-5189	Kineret	Recombinant human interleukin-1 receptor antagonist	153	17.26
Anifrolumab	D11082	761123	Saphnelo	Monoclonal Antibody	662	72.56
Ansuvimab	D11875	761172	Ebanga	Monoclonal Antibody	665	71.97
Antithrombin alfa	D08858	125284	Atryn	Antithrombin	432	49.04
Aprotinin	DB06692	20304	Trasylol	Hormone	58	6.52
Asfotase alfa	D10595	125513	Strensiq	Fusion protein	726	80.57
Asparaginase erwinia chrysanthemi	DB08886	125359	Erwinaze	Enzyme	327	35.05
Atezolizumab	DB11595	761034	Tecentriq	Monoclonal Antibody	662	72.30
Atoltivimab	D11468	761169	Inmazeb	Monoclonal Antibody	663	72.55
Avalglucosidase alfa	D11744	761194	Nexviazyme	Enzyme	896	99.37

(*Continued*)

Biosimilars Development Strategies

Name	Accession No.	BLA / NDA	Brand Name	Type of Molecule	AA#	MW
Avelumab	DB11945	761049	Bavencio	Monoclonal Antibody	666	71.91
Basiliximab	DB00074	103764	Simulect	Monoclonal Antibody	656	71.91
Becaplermin	DB00102	103691	Regranex	Growth factor	109	12.29
Belantamab mafodotin	D11594	761158	Blenrep	Monoclonal Antibody	664	72.94
Belatacept	DB06681	125288	Nulojix	Fusion protein	357	39.56
Belimumab	DB08879	125370	Benlysta	Monoclonal Antibody	449	47.68
Benralizumab	DB12023	761070	Fasenra	Monoclonal Antibody	665	73.03
Bevacizumab	DB00112	761231	Avastin	Monoclonal Antibody	667	73.28
Bezlotoxumab	D10453	761046	Zinplava	Monoclonal Antibody	664	72.78
Blinatumomab	DB09052	125557	Blincyto	Monoclonal Antibody	504	54.09
Brodalumab	6ZA31Y954Z	761032	Siliq	Monoclonal Antibody	656	72.03
Brolucizumab	D11083	761125	Beovu	Monoclonal Antibody	253	26.32
Burosumab	DB14012	761068	Crysvita	Monoclonal Antibody	660	72.04
Canakinumab	DB06168	125319	Ilaris	Monoclonal Antibody	662	72.59
Caplacizumab	DB06081	761112	Cablivi	Monoclonal Antibody	259	27.88
Catridecacog	D10532	125398	Tretten	Blood factor	732	83.27
Cemiplimab	DB14707	761097	Libtayo	Monoclonal Antibody	658	71.47
Cerliponase alfa	DB13173	761052	Brineura	Enzyme	544	59.31
Cetuximab	DB00002	125084	Erbitux	Monoclonal Antibody	663	72.72
Choriogonadotropin alfa	DB00097	21149	Ovidrel, Novarel	Hormone	237	25.72
Chorionic Gonadotropin (Human)	DB09126	17054	Novarel	Hormone	237	25.72
Chymopapain	DB06752	18663	Chymodiactin	Enzyme	352	39.41
Coagulation factor IX	DB13152	103249	Alphanine Sd, Beriplex, Immunine Vh, Kcentra, Octaplex	Blood factor	415	46.55

(Continued)

Name	Accession No.	BLA / NDA	Brand Name	Type of Molecule	AA#	MW
Coagulation Factor VIIa	DB00036	103665	Niastase RT, Novoseven, Sevenfact	Blood factor	406	45.08
Conestat alfa	D10845	125495	Ruconest	Inhibitors	478	52.84
Crizanlizumab	D11480	761128	Adakveo	Monoclonal Antibody	666	73.12
Daclizumab	DB00111	103749	Zenapax	Monoclonal Antibody	652	71.32
Daratumumab	DB09331	761036	Darzalex	Monoclonal Antibody	666	72.69
Darbepoetin alfa	DB00012	103951	Aranesp	Hormone	193	21.25
Denileukin diftitox	DB00004	103767	Ontak	Cytokine	521	57.65
Denosumab	DB06643	125320	Prolia, Xgeva	Monoclonal Antibody	667	72.58
Digoxin Immune Fab (Ovine)	DB00076	103141	Digibind	Monoclonal Antibody	437	47.30
Dinutuximab	D10559	125516	Unituxin	Monoclonal Antibody	663	72.49
Dornase alfa	DB00003	103532	Pulmozyme	Enzyme	255	28.65
Dostarlimab	DB15627	761174	Jemperli	Monoclonal Antibody	657	72.09
Drotrecogin alfa	DB00055	125029	Xigris	Recombinant activated human protein C	364	40.73
Dulaglutide	DB09045	125469	Trulicity	Fusion protein	275	29.84
Dupilumab	DB12159	761055	Dupixent	Monoclonal Antibody	670	73.45
Durvalumab	DB11714	761069	Imfinzi	Monoclonal Antibody	666	73.16
Ecallantide	DB05311	125277	Kalbitor	Inhibitors	60	7.06
Eculizumab	A3ULP0F556	125166	Soliris	Monoclonal Antibody	662	72.64
Efgartigimod alfa	DB15270	761195	Vyvgart	Inhibitors	454	51.27
Eflapegrastim	DB15001	761148	Rolvedon	Growth factor	616	68.41
Eftrenonacog Alfa	02E00T2QDE	125444	Alprolix	Fusion protein	867	97.38
Elosulfase alfa	DB09051	125460	Vimizim	Enzyme	496	55.41
Elotuzumab	DB06317	761035	Empliciti	Monoclonal Antibody	663	72.72

(Continued)

Name	Accession No.	BLA / NDA	Brand Name	Type of Molecule	AA#	MW
Emapalumab	3S252O2Z4X	761107	Gamifant	Monoclonal Antibody	670	72.67
Emicizumab	7NL2E3F6K3	761083	Hemlibra	Monoclonal Antibody	658	72.58
Eptinezumab	DB14040	761119	Vyepti	Monoclonal Antibody	660	71.60
Erenumab	DB14039	761077	Aimovig	Monoclonal Antibody	672	73.10
Erythropoietin	DB00016	125545	Epogen/ Procrit	Hormone	168	18.40
Etanercept	DB00005	761042	Erelzi	Fusion protein	467	51.24
Evinacumab	T8B2ORP1DW	761181	Evkeeza	Monoclonal Antibody	667	73.04
Evolocumab	D10557	125522	Repatha	Monoclonal Antibody	656	70.90
Filgrastim	DB00099	103353	Neupogen	Growth factor	175	18.80
Follitropin	DB00066	20582	Follistim	Hormone	203	22.67
Fremanezumab	PF8K38CG54	761089	Ajovy	Monoclonal Antibody	662	72.75
Galcaneuzumab	55KHL3P693	761063	Emgality	Monoclonal Antibody	659	72.04
Galsulfase	DB01279	125117	Naglazyme	Enzyme	497	56.01
Gemtuzumab ozogamicin	DB00056	761060	Mylotarg	Monoclonal Antibody	661	72.61
Glucarpidase	DB08898	125327	Voraxaze	Enzyme	415	44.02
Golimumab	91X1KLU43E	125289	Simponi	Monoclonal Antibody	671	73.47
Guselkumab	DB11834	761061	Tremfya	Monoclonal Antibody	664	71.92
Human C1- esterase inhibitor	P05155	125287	Berinert	Inhibitors	478	52.84
Hyaluronidase (Ovine)	DB00070	21640	Vitrase	Enzyme	476	54.19
Ibalizumab	LT369U66CE	761065	Trogarzo	Monoclonal Antibody	668	73.67
Ibritumomab tiuxetan	DB00078	125019	Zevalin	Monoclonal Antibody	652	71.70
Idarucizumab	DB09264	761025	Praxbind	Monoclonal Antibody	444	47.77
Idursulfase	DB01271	125151	Elaprase	Enzyme	525	59.30
Inebilizumab	74T7185BMM	761142	Uplizna	Monoclonal Antibody	668	73.18

(Continued)

Name	Accession No.	BLA / NDA	Brand Name	Type of Molecule	AA#	MW
Infliximab	B72HH48FLU	761086	Avsola	Monoclonal Antibody	440	47.75
Insulin aspart	DB01306	208751	Fiasp	Hormone	51	5.81
Insulin degludec	DB09564	203314	Tresiba	Hormone	50	5.69
Insulin detemir	DB01307	21536	Levemir	Hormone	50	5.69
Insulin glargine	DB00047	761215	Rezvoglar	Hormone	53	6.05
Insulin glulisine	DB01309	21629	Apidra	Hormone	51	5.81
Insulin lispro	DB00046	209196	Admelog	Hormone	51	5.80
Insulin regular	DB00030	19938	Novolin R	Hormone	51	5.80
Interferon alfa-2a	DB00034	103145/5098	Roferon-A	Cytokine	165	19.25
Interferon alfa-2b	DB00105	103132/ S-5202	Intron A	Cytokine	165	19.27
Interferon alfacon 1	DB00069	103663	Infergen	Cytokine	167	19.56
Interferon beta-1a	DB00060	103628/ S-5263	Avonex	Cytokine	166	20.03
Interferon beta-1b	DB00068	103471	Betaseron	Cytokine	165	19.88
Interferon gamma-1b	DB00033	103836	Actimmune	Cytokine	146	17.15
Ipilimumab	DB06186	125377	Yervoy	Monoclonal Antibody	663	72.69
Isatuximab	R30772KCU0	761113	Sarclisa	Monoclonal Antibody	664	72.61
Ixekizumab	DB11569	125521	Taltz	Monoclonal Antibody	664	73.09
L-asparaginase	DB00023	761179	Rylaze	Enzyme	348	36.85
Lanadelumab	DB14597	761090	Takhzyro	Monoclonal Antibody	664	72.86
Laronidase	DB00090	125058	Aldurazyme	Enzyme	626	69.90
Lepirudin	DB00001	NDA: 20807	Refludan	Inhibitors	65	6.99
Lixisenatide	DB09265	208471/S-005	Adlyxin	Hormone	44	4.86
Loncastuximab tersirine	7K5O7P6QIU	761196	Zynlonta	Monoclonal Antibody	660	72.23
Luspatercept-aamt	D11701	761136	Reblozyl	Enzyme	335	38
Lutropin alfa	DB00044	NDA: 21-322	Luveris, Pergoveris	Hormone	213	23.39
Maftivimab	KOP95331M4	761169	Inmazeb	Monoclonal Antibody	661	71.97
Margetuximab	K911R84KEW	761150	Margenza	Monoclonal Antibody	664	72.93
Mecasermin	DB01277	21839	Increlex	Hormone	70	7.65
Menotropins	DB00032	21663	Menopur	Hormone	416	46.05

(Continued)

Name	Accession No.	BLA / NDA	Brand Name	Type of Molecule	AA#	MW
Mepolizumab	90Z2UF0E52	125526	Nucala	Monoclonal Antibody	669	73.08
Metreleptin	DB09046	125390/S-024	Myalept	Hormone	147	16.16
Mirvetuximab soravtansine	DB12489	761310	Elahere	Monoclonal Antibody	665	72.85
Mogamulizumab	DB12498	761051	Poteligeo	Monoclonal Antibody	668	73.22
Muromonab	DB00075	103463	Orthoclone OKT3	Monoclonal Antibody	663	73.10
Natalizumab	3JB47N2Q2P	125104	Tysabri	Monoclonal Antibody	663	73.11
Naxitamab	9K8GNJ2874	761171	Danyelza	Monoclonal Antibody	660	72.22
Necitumumab	D10018	125547	Portrazza	Monoclonal Antibody	665	72.42
Nivolumab	DB09035	125554	Opdivo	Monoclonal Antibody	654	71.81
Obiltoxaximab	29Z5DNL48C	125509	Anthim	Monoclonal Antibody	663	72.76
Obinutuzumab	O43472U9X8	125486	Gazyva	Monoclonal Antibody	668	73.16
Ocrelizumab	A10SJL62JY	761053	Ocrevus	Monoclonal Antibody	665	72.91
Ocriplasmin	DB08888	125422	Jetrea	Enzyme	249	27.23
Odesivimab	UY9LQ8P6HW	761169	Inmazeb	Monoclonal Antibody	668	73.08
Ofatumumab	DB06650	125326	Arzerra, Kesimpta	Monoclonal Antibody	433	46.83
Olaratumab	D09939	761038	Lartruvo	Monoclonal Antibody	671	73.62
Olipudase alfa	DB12835	761261	Xenpozyme	Enzyme	570	63.65
Omalizumab	DB00043	103976	Xolair	Monoclonal Antibody	662	72.54
Oprelvekin	DB00038	103694	Neumega	Cytokine	177	19.05
Palifermin	DB00039	125103	Kepivance	Growth factor	140	16.28
Palivizumab	DQ448MW7KS	103770	Synagis	Monoclonal Antibody	227	24.93
Pancrelipase amylase	DB11065	20580	Cotazym	Enzyme	511	57.09
Panitumumab	6A901E312A	125147	Vectibix	Monoclonal Antibody	659	72.16
Parathyroid/ Preotact	DB05829	125511	Natpara	Hormone	84	9.42
Pembrolizumab	DB09037	125514	Keytruda	Monoclonal Antibody	665	73.14

(Continued)

Name	Accession No.	BLA / NDA	Brand Name	Type of Molecule	AA#	MW
Pertuzumab	DB06366	125409	Perjeta	Monoclonal Antibody	662	72.60
Polatuzumab vedotin	KG6VO684Z6	761121	Polivy	Monoclonal Antibody	665	72.63
Protein S human	DB13149	125421	Kcentra	Blood factor	676	75.12
Ramucirumab	DB05578	125477	Cyramza	Monoclonal Antibody	660	71.80
Ranibizumab	DB01270	761202	Byooviz	Monoclonal Antibody	445	48.37
Rasburicase	DB00049	103946	Elitek	Enzyme	301	34.11
Ravulizumab	C3VX249T6L	761108	Ultomiris	Monoclonal Antibody	662	72.61
Reslizumab	35A26E427H	761033	Cinqair	Monoclonal Antibody	657	71.91
Reteplase	DB00015	103786	Retavase	Enzyme	335	39.59
Rilonacept	DB06372	125249	Arcalyst	Fusion protein	880	####
Risankizumab	90ZX3Q3FR7	761105	Skyrizi	Monoclonal Antibody	663	72.80
Rituximab	DB00073	103705	Rituxan	Monoclonal Antibody	664	72.25
Romiplostim	DB05332	125268	Nplate	Growth factor	283	31.11
Romosozumab	3VHF2ZD92J	761062	Evenity	Monoclonal Antibody	663	72.94
Sacituzumab govitecan	M9BYU8XDQ6	761115	Trodelvy	Monoclonal Antibody	665	72.76
Sacrosidase	D05782	20772	Sucraid	Enzyme	513	58.63
Sargramostim	DB00020	103362/ S-5240	Leukine	Growth factor	127	14.43
Sarilumab	NU90V55F8I	761037	Kevzara	Monoclonal Antibody	660	72.06
Satralizumab	YB18NF020M	761149	Enspryng	Monoclonal Antibody	657	71.71
Sebelipase alfa	DB11563	125561	Kanuma	Enzyme	378	43
Secukinumab	DB09029	125504	Cosentyx	Monoclonal Antibody	672	73.97
Siltuximab	DB09036	125496	Sylvant	Monoclonal Antibody	662	72.49
Somatotropin recombinant	DB00052	761156	SOGROYA	Hormone	191	22.13
Tafasitamab	QQA9MLH692	761163	Monjuvi	Monoclonal Antibody	670	73.71
Tagraxofusp	DB14731	761116	Elzonris	Toxin	524	57.70
Taliglucerase alfa	D09675	22458	Elelyso	Enzyme	506	56.64
Tenecteplase	DB00031	103909	TNKase	Enzyme	527	58.78

(*Continued*)

Name	Accession No.	BLA / NDA	Brand Name	Type of Molecule	AA#	MW
Teprotumumab	Y64GQ0KC0A	761143	Tepezza	Monoclonal Antibody	663	72.82
Tezepelumab	RJ1IW3B4QX	761224	Tezspire	Monoclonal Antibody	662	72.30
Thyrotropin alfa	DB00024	20898	Thyrogen	Hormone	204	23.09
Tildrakizumab	DEW6X41BEK	761067	Ilumya	Monoclonal Antibody	660	72.22
Tocilizumab	DB06273	125276	Actemra	Monoclonal Antibody	662	72.54
Tositumomab	DB00081	125011	Bexxar	Monoclonal Antibody	657	71.94
Tralokinumab	GK1LYB375A	761180	Adbry	Monoclonal Antibody	663	72.06
Trastuzumab	DB00072	103792	Herceptin	Monoclonal Antibody	664	72.71
Urofollitropin	DB00094	21289	Bravelle	Hormone	203	22.67
Urokinase	DB00013	21846	Kinlytic	Enzyme	255	28.65
Ustekinumab	DB05679	125261	Stelara	Monoclonal Antibody	440	47.77
Vedolizumab	DB09033	125476	Entyvio	Monoclonal Antibody	670	73.42
Velaglucerase alfa	DB06720	22575	VPRIV	Enzyme	497	55.60
Vestronidase alfa	7XZ4062R17	761047	Mepsevii	Enzyme	629	72.56

NOTE

1 Administration FDAA. Biosimilars Product Information. https://www.fda.gov/drugs/biosimilars/biosimilar-product-information2024 [

2 Product Type and Selection Strategies

Generally, a developer would construct the facility for bacterial and mammalian cells; though mammalian cells are the most popular, the bacterial cells are having a comeback. However, the choice of product is best made by market competition, the CAPEX required to manufacture, and most importantly the regulatory approval cost that is primarily governed by the efficacy testing in patients. So, the advice to newcomers is to choose a product for which they are confident that the FDA will not need testing in patients. Over time, this will be a concession for all products but, until then, plan for the lowest investment product to begin.

2.1 BACKGROUND

Biologicals are mostly therapeutic recombinant proteins obtained by several different expression systems including mammalian cell lines, insects, and plants; new technological advancements are continuously being made to improve biological product expression. This investment is justified by the well-characterized genomes, plasmid vectors' versatility, availability of different host strains, and cost-effectiveness compared with other expression systems. There is an anticipation that within the next 5–10 years, up to 50% of all medicines in development will be biologicals.

The total number of biological entities approved by the FDA is 218, with multiple Biological License Application (BLAs) for some. The highest number of BLAs assigned are to somatropin, followed by albumin that was also the first BLA approved. Trend analysis shows that the trend for new biological entity approvals is turning significantly higher, albeit slower (Figure 2.1).

Antibodies dominate the biological drugs, soluble receptor constructs, immunoglobulin fusion proteins, and secreted naturally occurring proteins. The most prominent examples are tumor necrosis factor (TNF) alpha-blocking antibodies (infliximab and adalimumab) and the soluble TNF receptor fusion protein (etanercept) for the treatment of rheumatoid arthritis, the anti-CD20 antibody rituximab for non-Hodgkin's lymphoma, the anti-vascular endothelial growth factor A (VEGF-A) antibody bevacizumab for colorectal and other cancers, and the anti-human epidermal growth factor receptor 2 (HER2) antibody trastuzumab for the treatment of breast cancer.

Beyond these "classical" drugs, the biologics space has grown fast over recent years. For example, by introducing antibody-small molecular weight drug conjugates or bispecific antibodies, this trend will grow fast in the coming years.

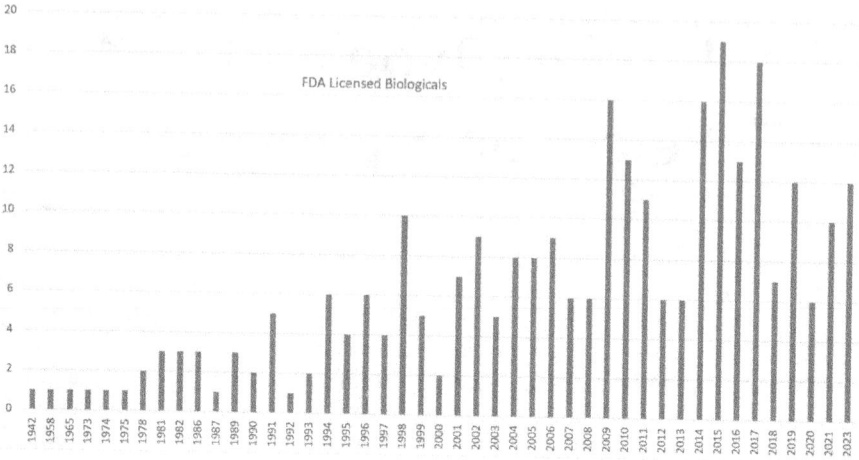

FIGURE 2.1   BLAs licensed by the FDA from 12 to November 2023. Source: FDA.

2.2   EXCLUSIVITY

Biological products can obtain market exclusivity from a combination of three primary sources: (i) regulatory exclusivities, (ii) patents, and (iii) trade secrets or proprietary information. Regulatory Exclusivities and Patents protect a product's market for a defined period. The Biological Price Competition and Innovation Act (BPCIA) provides 12 years of regulatory exclusivity to innovative biologic products approved by filing a full BLA. United States patents have a "twenty-year term" that begins on the date the patent issues and ends on the date that is 20 years from the earliest priority date the application was filed (There is an exception to the "twenty-year term," which applies to patents that were in force on June 8, 1995, or that issued from an application that was filed before June 8, 1995. Patents within this category have a term that is the greater of the "twenty-year term" or 17 years from the patent grant date (35 USC 154 (c)). However, some of the baseline periods of exclusivities defined in the statutory provision can be extended for additional periods by pediatric exclusivities, patent term extension, and patent term adjustments.

Regulatory exclusivities provide market protection to innovative products regardless of whether the products have patent protection. In the absence of patent protection, a generic drug can immediately enter the market upon the expiration of the regulatory exclusivity period. Therefore, creating and managing a strong patent portfolio is a crucial element of the business model for biopharmaceutical companies.

To balance competition and innovation, the BPCIA established two periods of exclusivity applicable to a brand-name biologic (i.e., the reference product)—one with a duration of 4 years and the other with a duration of 12 years. Periods of regulatory exclusivity attach upon approval or licensure of a drug or biologic, respectively, if certain statutory requirements are met, limiting competitors' ability to reference the data generated by brand-name drug manufacturers.

During the 4-year exclusivity period, a BLA for a proposed biological or inter-changeable product referencing the brand-name biologic may not be submitted to the FDA. During the 12-year exclusivity period, a BLA's approval for a proposed biologi-cal or interchangeable product referencing the brand-name biologic may not be made effective. This means that FDA may not approve a BLA for a proposed biological or interchangeable product until 12 years after the date on which the reference product was first licensed, and a BLA for a proposed biological or interchangeable product cannot be submitted to the FDA until 4 years after the date on which the reference product was licensed.

Certain biologics are not eligible for the reference product exclusivity, for exam-ple, if an application is for a minor change to a previously licensed biologic. A new biologic may be eligible for an additional 6-month period of exclusivity that would attach to the 12- and 4-year periods if the developer conducts pediatric studies according to a written request from the FDA. Additionally, a biologic approved to treat a rare disease or condition may be granted 7 years of orphan drug exclusivity for the protected indication, in which case the FDA may not license another biologic for the protected orphan indication until after the expiration of the 7- or 12-year exclu-sivity period, whichever is later. While the first biological for a brand name is not eligible for exclusivity, the first interchangeable product is. This means that the FDA will not make an interchangeability determination for a subsequent biologic relying on the same reference product for any condition of use until such exclusivity expires. The periods of exclusivity available for biological products under the Federal Food, Drug, and Cosmetic Act (PHSA) are generally longer than those for chemical drugs under the Federal Food, Drug, and Cosmetic Act (FFDCA) (i.e., 5-year new chemical entity exclusivity and 3-year new clinical study exclusivity).

While the FDA is not required by law to publish information about approved bio-logics and biologicals, the agency does so voluntarily with the Purple Book's publica-tion. Unlike the Orange Book, which is available in paper form and as a searchable, electronic database, the Purple Book consists of two lists—one for biological prod-ucts (including proposed biological and interchangeable products) licensed by Center for Drug Evaluation and Research (CDER) and the other for those licensed by Center for Biologicals Evaluation and Research (CBER). For brand-name biologics, the list identifies the date the biologic was licensed (i.e., approved). If the FDA evaluated the product for reference product exclusivity, the exclusivity would expire.

Patents can be issued at any point during the development cycle of a drug product. For example, some patents claiming the drug substance itself may be issued before or during the NDA or BLA filing. Other patents, such as a patent that claims the commercial formulation or the use of a customized delivery device, or a detailed treatment regimen, will likely be issued much later after human clinical testing is completed. Also, life cycle management practices will occasionally give rise to sub-marine patents that provide an unexpected patent exclusivity extension.

A submarine patent is a term used to refer to a patent that was filed before the change in the law in 1995 but issued years later due to a delay, such as an interference proceeding. The patent application remains secret in the patent office because it was filed before the requirement to publish the application and then suddenly surfaces, hence submarine. The result is a patent that is issued years after the technology has advanced, and the patent receives a term of 17 years from the issue because it is issued under the rules of the previous statute.

Furthermore, innovation is an inherent feature of product development and later discovered inventions, such as an optimized purification process or method of use, could provide additional patent exclusivity in the form of a late issuing patent. Therefore, the regulatory market and the patent exclusivities may, or may not, run concurrently.

Trade secret laws can vary from state to state but share the unifying characteristics of requiring that the information is of economic value to the owner. The owner establishes and maintains reasonable efforts to protect the information from public disclosure.

Typically, subject matter that a biopharmaceutical manufacturer considers to be proprietary trade secrets is not included in their patent disclosures, which are subject to publication.

Trade secret protection is not limited by any defined statutory period and can provide companies with a competitive advantage for as long as the information remains confidential. For example, the biologic manufacturer could keep information about critical process controls used during manufacturing or downstream bioprocess steps to produce the reference product. As long as the information remains confidential, the trade secret/proprietary information will confer the manufacturer a competitive advantage. Manufacturing process controls are developed and established for each product/process and play an integral role in defining the biological drug product's quality and purity.

A single biological product can be protected by numerous patents claiming subject matter ranging from nucleic acid and amino acid sequences, expression vectors, cell-based expression systems, upstream and downstream methods for producing and purifying the drug substance, optimized formulations developed to stabilize the drug product, devices used for administration, general methods of use, indication-specific methods of use, functional assays developed to release the drug product for sale, elucidate the method of action, and analytical or diagnostic assays. Given the patentable subject matter scope, it is not uncommon to identify anywhere from 50 to more than 100 patent filings relevant to a single biological product. Table 7.4 highlights the possible patent claims available in the case of an antibody product.

It was only in 1978 that the US patent 4,082,613 claimed a method producing insulin genetically modified fungal cells; in 1980, came Cohen patent (US 4,237,224) that claimed a process for producing biologically functional molecular chimeras and in 1983, Axel (4,399,216) claimed a process of inserting DNA into eucaryotic cells and for producing proteinaceous materials. A new era of biological medicines thus opened. All these pivotal patents have expired but the race to patent new genes, manufacturing process, formulations, routes of administration, and indications continues creating a nightmare for biosimilar developers once the gene patents expire, to develop a biosimilar product—a primary reason for the delayed adoption of biosimilars in the USA (Table 2.1).

Figure 2.2 shows the number of patents awarded to selected biological drugs.

TABLE 2.1
Possible Patent Claims for Antibody Products

Antibody Product	Possible Patent Claims
Amino Acid Sequence	Amino Acid sequence of: Complete Heavy and Light Chains Heavy and Light Chain Variable Regions CDR regions Modifications made to the framework, CDR, or Fc regions
Nucleic Acid Sequence	Nucleic acid sequences encoding any or all of the above-listed amino acid sequences
Expression Vector	Every individual element and/or combination of the vector elements is used to express the sequence in a suitable host cell, including promoter, enhancer, other regulatory sequences, and selection marker.
Expression System	Host Cells engineered to express the product
Culture Conditions	Media Components Culture Method/Feed Media Optimized Culture conditions
Purification	Chromatography Methods claiming the use of particular resins alone or in series Optimized Conditions Compositions having a defined level of purity or homogeneity
Formulation	Pharmaceutical compositions comprising the drug product
Device	Device for administration and use thereof
Methods of Use	Broad mechanism-based methods of use Disease-specific methods of use Indication-specific treatment regimens corresponding to the product label
Diagnostic Methods and Kits	Methods and/or kits used to identify select patents that are more or less likely to respond to treatment
Analytical Methods	Assays developed to monitor the quality or purity of the product
Platform Technology	Platform technologies and assays used to discover or optimize the structural and/or functional features of the product or processes used to manufacture or purify the product

2.3 FORMULATION

Additionally, while injections predominantly delivered the first biologicals, it is anticipated that future products may be given by routes such as oral, dermatological, and inhaled formulations based on a variety of encapsulation approaches aiming to minimize the biologic instability caused by protein aggregation and denaturation because of physicochemical modifications such as deamination, hydrolysis, and oxidation, among others.

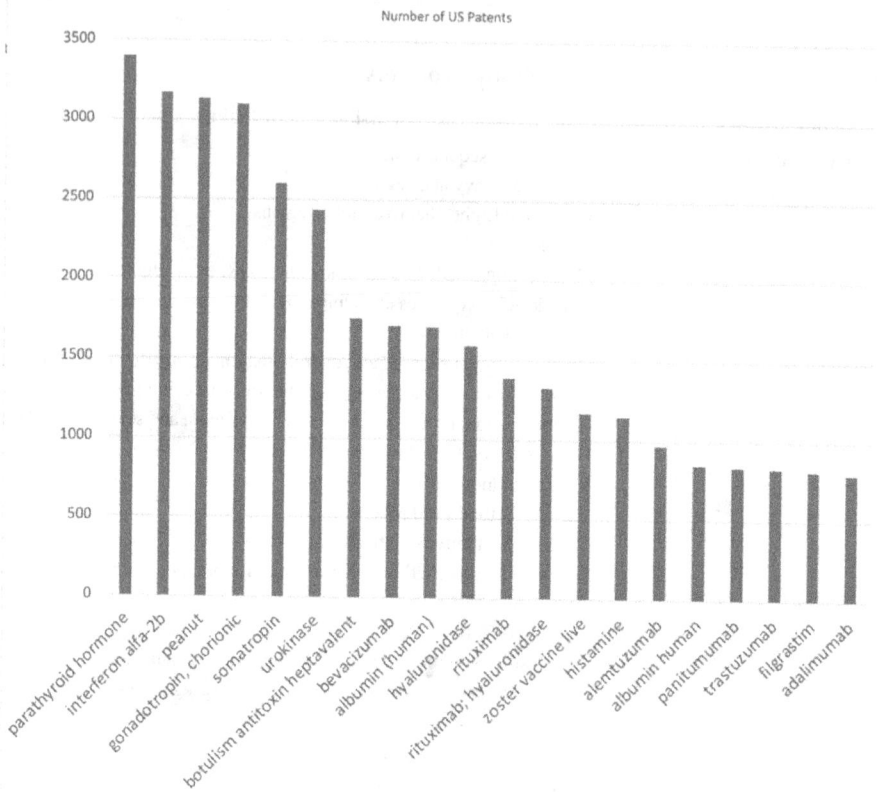

FIGURE 2.2 Number of patents awarded to biological molecules—top candidates.

The formulation of biologicals is a broad field of study with several peculiarities compared to small molecule drugs.

First, most protein drugs are administered by parenteral routes, and, as a result, most of the science of protein drug formulation deals with the art of injectable formulations. The choice of delivery route is restricted because of (i) the instability of the protein structures in many sites of administration environment, such as the acidity in the gastrointestinal tract, (ii) the large molecular size and high hydrophilicity preventing absorption across some biological membranes, leading to faster elimination, and (iii) high dose-response sensitivity that does not allow significant variation in the bioavailability.

Second, there are several common structural features of proteins, such as (i) functional groups methionine, cysteine, histidine, tryptophan, and tyrosine, all of which are subject to oxidation, requiring some common approaches to stabilize, (ii) conformational changes, and aggregation, properties peculiar to large molecules, requiring the inclusion of product-specific formulation components to prevent aggregation, and (iii) inactive components having a greater impact on the bioavailability and conversion to more immunogenic forms with a possibility of altered pharmacokinetic profile that may change the effectiveness of the drug.

Third, all proteins are sensitive to temperature, light, and agitation during storage, shipping, and handling. In some instances, the label includes a caution not to shake the product. With so many variables that can affect the quality and efficacy, the formulation challenges are heightened to address many aspects not generally considered in small molecule drugs.

Biologicals' formulations largely vary depending on the delivery route, which is mostly parenteral, but new advances are extending the routes to many other non-invasive routes. The choice of administration route is made based on the practicality and probability factors requiring a detailed understanding of the interaction of biologicals with the environment of the route of administration. Over the past two decades, many computation tools have become available that allow the fast creation of decision matrices to optimize the formulations.

Each route of administration faces unique biological barriers due to the site of administration's anatomical and physiological characteristics. Many formulation approaches have been developed to overcome these barriers, including the advances in information technology, biotechnology, and nanotechnology, combined with sophisticated medical devices, electric or magnetic forces, or sonic waves to maximize non-invasive drug effectiveness delivery systems.

A formulation is intended to deliver a biological active to the site of administration, from where it crosses biological barriers, entering the bloodstream, and finally, the site of action that may or may not is known. Given the high likelihood of the degradation of products during the shelf-life, a large volume of proprietary technology has been developed, including thousands of patents, to enable a dosage form to deliver the drug to the site of action.

Since biologicals' development is costly, scientists inevitably get engaged with the evaluation of the intellectual property relating to biological manufacturing and delivery system. Chapter 8 provides details about intellectual property and its management and forms a required reading for the scientists engaged in the formulation of biologicals.

The formulation composition of biologicals, like other products, depends on the route of administration and the physicochemical properties of the product. However, the high molecular mass and the large size of drug molecules result in poor membrane permeability, limiting the choice of delivery routes. For example, drugs with a relatively small molecular mass of <500 Da readily penetrate through membranes in the gastrointestinal tract and the skin through passive diffusion. Concerning ocular delivery, the human retina restricts the diffusion of macromolecules >76 kDa due to inner and outer plexiform layers, and macromolecules above 150 kDa are unable to reach the inner retina. The nasal mucosa also exhibits low membrane permeability for molecules larger than 1 kDa. Given that proteins >3–5 kDa are generally regarded as peptidyl molecules and antibodies with a mass of 150 kDa, the hydrophilicity of biologicals obviates several routes of administration.

Most protein drugs are highly hydrophilic with a log P value of less than zero, which hampers drug permeation across biological membranes and creates challenges with respect to the delivery of protein drugs to intracellular targets (See Appendix of the chapter). Due to the lipophilic nature of biological membranes and the paracellular space, which is 3–10 Å, the large size and hydrophilic nature of proteins limit their diffusion and passage through paracellular pathways. Therefore, the cellular uptake of hydrophilic proteins is primarily controlled by active transport or endocytosis rather than passive diffusion. For proteins, one of the major disadvantages of the endocytic pathway is entrapment by endosomes, which eventually leads to degradation by lysosomal enzymes.

Another physicochemical drug property influencing absorption is the surface charge of a biological, which is derived from the amino acid sequence of the protein and its surroundings' pH. This physicochemical property is complex and heterogeneous; it is typically caused by deamination, isomerization, or post-translational modification, leading to a change in the net charge of a protein and acidic formation and basic variants. The surface charge can cause protein drugs to interact with molecules on the cell surfaces or tissue components, thereby affecting the absorption, distribution, and elimination of proteins in the body.

2.3.1 HIGHER CONCENTRATION FORMULATIONS

Biosimilars need not have the same formulation as the reference product, giving a lot of latitude to development; while it is preferred for the biosimilar product not to innovate the formulation, it may often be necessary due to patent issues or cost considerations.

High concentrations are often needed to accommodate the low management volume combined with their practical applications for subcutaneous administration. Sadly, with growing protein concentrations, the physical behavior of such a substance will change dramatically. Such properties may include substantially improving opalescence, viscosity, and protein aggregation/immunogenicity of the solution. Such altered properties challenge processes for the manufacture of drug products, product administration, and marketability.

Treatments with high doses of more than 1 mg/kg or 100 mg per dose often allow formulations to be formulated at concentrations exceeding 100 mg/mL due to the small volume (<1.5 mL) that the subcutaneous routes may provide. Achieving these high-concentration formulations is a developmental challenge for proteins that have the potential to accumulate at higher concentrations. Even for the intravenous delivery route where large quantities can be managed.

The interaction between proteins at higher concentration formulation may result in reversible self-association, which may further progress toward the formation of insoluble aggregates; at a higher concentration, the probability of one molecule bumping into other increases, enhancing the probability of formation of reversible oligomers such as a dimer, tetramers, etc. The formation of aggregates occurs through multiple mechanisms, including the formation of covalent linkages (e.g., disulfide exchange). Even minor conformational changes in the native structure may lead to the formation of aggregates. The probability of such an occurrence is greater in higher concentrations.

High concentration is defined by the solution where the solutes occupy a significant portion of the solution (≥0.1). Another description of a high-concentration solution is the situation where the molecular size and the distance between the Van der Waals' surfaces are of the same magnitude. Regardless of the meaning, high concentration refers to the molecular proximity intermolecular space. The primary challenge in achieving high-concentration formulation is the solubility of the target protein. Solubility is controlled by its molecular property (sequence, charge distribution, etc.) as well as by the solution condition, such as pH, ionic strength, excipient concentration, etc. The solubility of a protein is defined by the maximum amount of the protein present in a solution, without the appearance of any visible aggregates, precipitates, etc. A more technical definition will be the maximum amount of protein that remains in the solution, following 30 minutes of centrifugation at 30,000 g in the presence of co-solute. Besides solubility, there are other issues associated with the development of high-concentration mAb formulation. These include opalescence, viscosity, and aggregation. Opalescence is commonly expressed by the turbidity unit with nephelometry. Although opalescence is not a major issue and may occur independently of aggregation, it remains a major concern as it may fail to satisfy patient compliance due to its appearance. Reversible protein–protein and liquid–liquid phase separation may also lead to opalescence. Protein–protein interaction at high concentration is a significant factor that may influence opalescence and viscosity. When molecules are near, they can interact with each other, resulting in reversible self-association and an increase in viscosity, opalescence, and even aggregation.

The increase in viscosity at high concentrations has a significant impact on manufacturability and injectability. Tangential flow filtration is one of the leading technologies used for buffer exchange and concentrating proteins during large-scale manufacturing (clinical and commercial). The increase in viscosity at high concentration may create back pressure high enough to exceed the pump's capacity inducing considerable stress to the mAb, as rapid pumping and continuous circulation through the narrow tubing create significant cavitation and shear stress. The increase in viscosity may further increase the backpressure that can be more destabilizing to the protein. At a minimum, this increases the processing time, and in turn, the cost of manufacture. The increase in viscosity has a significant impact on the administration of subcutaneous dosage form. The glide force describes the ease of subcutaneous injection or extrusion force, which refers to the force required to push the liquid through the syringe. While there are various factors, including needle gauge and the needle's length, associated with glide force, one of the main contributing factors is solution viscosity. Viscosity has been reported to be directly correlated to glide force for subcutaneous injection. The increase in viscosity increases the injection site and the pain at the injection site, leading to decreased patient compliance.

One of the latest emerging concepts for addressing protein stability and high viscosity issues is the formation of "nanoclusters"—densely packed protein molecules formed in the presence of a crowder such as trehalose. Protein molecules were shown to be crowded into colloidally stable dispersions of distinct nanoclusters (35–80 nm), exhibiting hydrodynamic diameters of equilibrium at very high concentrations (up to 320 mg/mL), without gelation. An IgG protein's nanoclusters are in harmony with monomers, which can be less than 2%. One dispersion of the nanocluster at 220 mg/mL in the presence of 70 mg/trehalose showed a viscosity of 36 cP, which is syringeable through a 25 G needle. Subcutaneous injection of these preparations for nanoclusters resulted in indistinguishable pharmacokinetics against a standard solution for the antibody in mice.

It is conceivable that the distances between protein molecules in nanoclusters are smaller than those in the bulk solution. The shorter distance could enhance protein–protein interactions and potentially lead to stability issues. The nanocluster concept is relatively new and needs further evaluation.

2.3.2   LIQUID FORMULATIONS

Liquid formulations require the study of electrostatic interactions, Van der Waals interactions, hydrogen bonding, and hydrophobicity. For example, the native conformation of biologics can be stabilized by high concentrations of saccharides such as sucrose, trehalose, lactose, etc., as well as by polyhydrated alcohols such as sorbitol, mannitol, polyethylene glycol, etc. due to the preferential exclusion from the protein surface, thus providing stabilization. Saccharose is excluded because of increased surface tension. The solubility of proteins can often be increased by adding small concentrations of salt, a phenomenon called "salting in." Salts are also used as tonicity modifiers; however, in some cases, it may negatively impact conformational stability. So, the option of counterions (referring to the Hofmeister series) and their concentration can be used to modify the biological's stability profile. In preformulation screening, this is considered critical. For example, the same pH condition can be obtained with different buffer species at different concentrations (i.e., at different ionic strengths) and can thus modify the protein's stability. Ligand binding may also support the native protein state, as seen, for example, by binding Zn^{2+} to the growth hormone in humans.

Surface-active agents are often used to prevent the adsorption, denaturation, and aggregation of proteins at interfaces (both air–water and solid–water) and affect stability by differential binding to the protein's native or denatured states. Agitation and freeze-thaw stress experiments are often used to demonstrate surface denaturation mechanisms and the addition of low surfactant concentrations such as Polysorbate 20, Polysorbate 80, Pluronic F68, or others can be effective in minimizing both soluble and insoluble aggregates. Leachates such as metal ions, barium from glass vials, vulcanizing agents from stoppers, tungsten oxide from prefilled syringes, and silicone oil penetration are additional concerns related to the primary contact surfaces that need to be addressed during excipient selection. For example, EDTA can be used for removing metal leachates from stoppers. So, the option of counterions (referring to the Hofmeister series) and their concentration can be used to modify the biological's stability profile. This is considered critical during screening before formulation. For example, the same pH state can be obtained with different buffer species at different concentrations (i.e., at different ionic strengths) and can alter protein stability. Ligand binding, as seen, for example, with the binding of Zn^{2+} to human growth hormone, can also support the native state of proteins.

One-third of biological products are available as multidose, and these typically require antimicrobial preservatives to be added. By inducing protein aggregation, the preservatives may present additional stabilization challenges for biologicals. The common preservatives include m-cresol, benzyl alcohol or phenol, phenoxyethanol, and chlorobutanol. Screening of different preservatives is recommended before use, either alone or in combination.

2.3.3 Lyophilized Formulations

Lyophilization with appropriate excipients may improve protein stability against aggregation by decreasing protein mobility and restricting conformational flexibility with the added benefit of minimizing hydrolytic reactions consequent to water removal. The addition of suitable excipients, including lyoprotectants, can prevent aggregates' formation during the lyophilization process and final product storage. A key parameter for effective protection is the molar ratio of the lyoprotectant to the protein. Generally, molar ratios of 300:1 or greater are required to provide suitable stability, especially for room-temperature storage. Such ratios can also, however, lead to an undesirable increase in viscosity.

The instability of protein in an aqueous solution without preservatives may require lyophilization. Aligning the desired requirements for stability, storage, and shipping with the target product profile makes lyophilization an essential alternative to a liquid formulation, especially for highly thermolabile products and live virus vaccine products. The lyophilization process requires freezing, followed by primary and secondary drying under vacuum; the drying process itself presents a new set of challenges. Denaturation can occur during freezing, either in the freeze-concentrate state, frozen surface interfaces, or through cold denaturation. Formulations should also address the impact of local salt and buffer concentrations and increase the concentration of trapped oxygen during the freeze-concentrate process.

Similarly, changes in pH due to buffer crystallization have to be considered for lyophilized products during the formulation design space. For example, buffering at physiological pH conditions with a low concentration (including 10mM) of potassium phosphate over sodium phosphate buffer is preferable; this can be due to the pH change as a function of increasing buffer concentration and a large pH shift during freezing for sodium phosphate. Due to minimal pH changes during freezing, citrate, Tris, and Histidine are good choices for the buffer if at the correct pH range. Likewise, antioxidants (e.g., ascorbates) and scavengers (e.g., thiourea) may be added for the reduction of oxidation.

External stabilizers known as lyoprotectants may be required in addition to cryoprotectants. Liquid pre-formulation screening, for example, could suggest that sorbitol is a good stabilizer; however, sorbitol is not preferred in dried formulations because of its low glass transition temperature. It should be noted that the two key attributes of lyoprotectants are high glass transition temperatures to reduce molecular mobility while maintaining the native state in the dried state by acting as a strong water replacement (e.g., sucrose and trehalose). Therefore, the use of reduced sugars (e.g., lactose) must be specifically measured in the risk assessment analysis. Nevertheless, the possibility of phase separation (especially for a multi-stabilizer system) can limit some combinations of excipients (for example, PEG-Dextran). Likewise, low pH acid hydrolysis capacity makes trehalose a better option for sucrose.

Bulking agents are also added to the lyophilized product to avoid product "blowout" for products with a low concentration (including 1% solid). Excipients can function as amorphous bulking agents (e.g., sucrose, trehalose, lactose, raffinose, dextran, hydroxyethyl starch (HES), or as crystalline bulking agents (e.g., glycine and mannitol) for amorphous excipients (such as HES) or high eutectic temperatures (T_{eu})

for crystalline excipients (such as glycine and mannitol). Nonetheless, the presence of mannitol hydrate form and the risk of glass breakage during manufacture (be it due to high fill volume, incorrect freezing procedure, and/or high concentration) can restrict mannitol selection during excipient screening.

Administration, reducing pain when given, may be beneficial. Isotonicity of a lyophile is difficult to achieve due to the concentration of both the protein and the excipients during the reconstitution cycle. Excipient: 500:1 protein molar ratio may result in hypertonic preparations if the protein is targeted at >100 mg/mL.

While freeze-drying is one of the most widely used processes for protein drugs, this method has several disadvantages, and several alternative drying methods are developed that include spray-drying, spray-freezing, supercritical drying of fluids, supercritical fluid drying, and foam drying applied to proteins including insulin, trypsin, human growth hormones, and monoclonal antibodies.

2.4   ROUTE OF ADMINISTRATION

Every administration route has its limitations depending on the anatomical size and position, microclimate, specific physiological conditions, and formulations. The volume and viscosity of the fluid in the rectum may also affect drug absorption.

The pH conditions in various biological environments can affect the ionization, chemical instability, and absorption of protein-based drugs and their delivery systems. For example, protein drugs are often unstable at physiological pH. Notably, the strongly acidic gastric environment (pH 1–3) causes destabilization of protein drugs in the stomach, but chemical degradation reduces significantly in the ileum and colon due to higher pH. In an ocular delivery system, the buffering agent plays a vital role since hyperosmotic solutions cause transient dehydration of the anterior chamber tissues, while hypotonic solutions may cause edema.

2.4.1   Intravenous

The most common routes to deliver biopharmaceutics include intravenous bolus, intravenous infusion, and subcutaneous. Most drugs that would have either low or highly variable bioavailability are administered by the intravenous route to assure exact dosing, like oncology drugs. Intravenous injections are also preferred for drugs that might irritate subcutaneous tissue. However, this route cannot be recommended for self-administration of drugs, a significant cost element of drug therapy. There are not many formulation concerns except that the drug must be either in a solution form or in an extremely fine emulsion to prevent veins blockage. Recently, some biologicals that were initially developed as intravenous injection or infusion have been reformulated for subcutaneous administration to enable self-administration.

2.4.2   Subcutaneous

The first biological, insulin, was approved as a subcutaneous product. Intravenous bolus or infusion is the common route for drugs where a dose must be calculated, such as in the use of oncology drugs administered by professionals. However, recently, there is a shift taking place from intravenous to subcutaneous administration for

TABLE 2.2

Examples of Biologicals Delivered in Subcutaneous Dosage Forms

Molecule	Brand Name (Originator)	Dosing Frequency	Injection Volume	Device
Abatacept	Orencia (Bristol-Myers Squibb)	q1w	1 mL	Prefilled syringe, prefilled pen/autoinjector
Adalimumab	Humira (AbbVie)	q2w	0.4–0.8 mL	Prefilled syringe, vial, prefilled pen
Anakinra	Kineret (Swedish Orphan Biovitrum GmbH)[a]	q1d or q2d	0.67 mL	Prefilled syringe
Certolizumab pegol	Cimzia (UCB-Euronext and BEL20)[a]	q2w and q4w	1 mL	Prefilled syringe, vial, prefilled pen
Etanercept	Enbrel (Amgen)	q1w or twice weekly	0.5–1 mL	Prefilled syringe, vial, prefilled pen/autoinjector, prefilled cartridge for reusable autoinjector
Glatiramer acetate	Copaxone (Teva)	q1d or three times per week	1 mL	Prefilled syringe, pen/autoinjector
Golimumab	Simponi (Janssen)	q1m	0.5–1 mL	Prefilled syringe, prefilled pen/autoinjector
Insulin	Several	PRN	Variable	Vials, prefilled pen, syringes
Interferon-beta-1a	Rebif (EMD Serono/Pfizer)	Three times per week	0.2–0.5 mL	Prefilled syringe, prefilled pen/autoinjector, electronic injection system
Interferon beta-1b	Betaseron/ Betaferon (Bayer)	q2d	0.25–1 mL	Prefilled syringe. vial, autoinjector
Interferon beta-1b	Extavia (Novartis)	q2d	0.25–1 mL	Prefilled syringe, vial, autoinjector
Peg-interferon beta-1a	Plegridy (Biogen)	q2w	0.5 mL	Prefilled syringe, prefilled pen/autoinjector
Rituximab	MabThera/Rituxan Hycela (Roche)	q3w–q3mc	11.7–13.4 mL	Vial and syringe
Sarilumab	Kevzara (Sanofi-Aventis)	q2w	1.14 mL	Prefilled syringe, prefilled pen
Tocilizumab	Actemra (Roche)	q1w and q2w	0.9 mL	Prefilled syringe, prefilled pen
Trastuzumab	Herceptin (Roche)	q3w	5 mL	Vial and syringe

economic reasons. After subcutaneous formulations of trastuzumab and rituximab introduced in Europe in 2013 and 2014, respectively, several drugs were reformulated as subcutaneous dosage forms shifting from intravenous, allowing self-injection rheumatoid arthritis, multiple sclerosis, or primary immunodeficiency therapies, where mixed dosing (not calculated based on body weight) is recommended (Table 2.2).

The biological product pharmacokinetic profile administered through the subcutaneous route is distinct from that of the intravenous form. A biotherapeutic intravenous infusion or injection directly into the bloodstream usually results in immediate maximum serum concentrations (C_{max}), whereas the pharmacokinetic profile of biological products subcutaneously injected is typically characterized by a sluggish rate of absorption from the subcutaneous extracellular matrix with C_{max} levels below those achieved with intravenous dosing. This pattern of absorption of macromolecules into the blood results from their reduced permeability across the vascular endothelial; hence, lymphatics provide an alternative pathway of absorption into the circulation system. Nonetheless, lymphatic absorption has also been identified as a barrier to the full infiltration of molecules injected subcutaneously. Such factors that may contribute to the incomplete bioavailability of subcutaneously injected molecules may include the dose formulation structure, duration, pH, viscosity, interactions with interstitial glycosaminoglycans, and proteins and enzymatic degradation.

Following subcutaneous injection, molecules reach the systemic circulation via either the blood capillaries or the lymphatic system. Unlike small molecules, biological products with molecular weights of >20 kDa exhibit limited transport into the blood capillaries and cross into the circulation system predominantly via the lymphatics. Such increased exposure to the lymphatic system has led to the suggestion that biotherapeutic subcutaneous administration may be more immunogenic than intravenous dosing. In this context, it is necessary to consider the production of anti-drug antibodies with the various routes of administration per se and their effect on the biotherapeutic's exposure, efficacy, and safety. The regulatory agencies currently require immunogenicity testing of the subcutaneous dosage form over intravenous if there is an option.

A drawback of subcutaneous administration of biological products is the incomplete bioavailability of the injected molecule, ranging widely from 50% to 80% for mAbs and even more for other biological products. As for the enzymes involved and their translation through organisms, the underlying pre-systemic catabolism at the subcutaneous administration site or the lymphatic system is still poorly understood. For mAbs, subcutaneous bioavailability appears to be inversely correlated with clearance after intravenous dosing, so that mAbs with a lower intravenous clearance exhibit higher subcutaneous bioavailability. This correlation may be due to hematopoietic cells (e.g., macrophages or dendritic cells) in both subcutaneous first-pass clearance and systemic clearance after intravenous dosing. Since inadequate bioavailability typically leads to the need for a higher dose for subcutaneous infusions than for intravenous infusions, the cost of goods for subcutaneous formulations may be more significant.

To increase the subcutaneous bioavailability of a biotherapeutic, subcutaneous infusions can be co-administered (or produced as coformulations) with the dispersion-enhancer hyaluronidase. This enzyme facilitates the spreading of an injected fluid in the subcutaneous tissue. This increased dispersion in the interstitial tissue can result in higher bioavailability of a co-injected molecule.

Subcutaneous injections are often formulated in a buffered aqueous solution, some of which can be irritating like the citrate buffer. In an interesting example, the best-selling biological drug, Humira, was launched in a citrate buffer that causes smarting upon injection; once the patent on the gene sequence expired, Abbvie reformulated the product by removing the buffer and justified it by stating that the large proteins themselves have a buffering effect. Therefore, there is no need for a citrate buffer. The new formulation is more concentrated, reducing the injection volume, less irritation, and allowed Abbvie another patent that now protects the product for decades. Some sustained-release subcutaneous therapeutics have been available for several decades, such as insulin glargine that precipitates subcutaneous injection to allow prolonged release. Recent advances in polymer science have led to hydrogels that provide sustained drug release, have high tissue biocompatibility, and allow self-administration by the patient. Hydrogels provide a deformable drug depot that slowly elutes a high drug concentration to surrounding tissue for an extended period. However, because most hydrogels only physically incorporate, instead of forming covalent bonds to the drugs, a rapid drug release occurs over a few hours to days, limiting their value for sustained drug delivery.

2.4.3 PULMONARY

Many drugs under development for pulmonary delivery include interleukin-1 receptor (asthma therapy), heparin (blood clotting), human insulin (diabetes), alpha-1 antitrypsin (emphysema and cystic fibrosis), interferons (multiple sclerosis and hepatitis B and C), and calcitonin and other peptides (osteoporosis). Inhalation delivery methods may apply gene therapy via tissue targeting and organ targeting. Inhale's novel dry powder formulation, processing, and filling, combined with aerosol device technology, will provide many patients who previously received injections with the ability to inhale medicine independently and painlessly into the deep lung, where it will be absorbed into the bloodstream naturally and efficiently.

The delivery device plays a critical role in the effectiveness of pulmonary drug administration; thus, selecting a delivery device is essential in the formulation design for pulmonary drug delivery. The most used devices used to deliver therapeutics as aerosols are nebulizers (e.g., jet nebulizers, ultrasonic nebulizers, and vibrating mesh nebulizers), metered-dose inhalers, and dry powder inhalers.

Various nanotechnology-based formulation approaches have been extensively examined for effective protein delivery via the pulmonary route. In general, nanoparticles appear to be promising as a pulmonary delivery carrier of proteins due to their targeting capability and controlled drug release. Also, nanoparticles <200 nm in size might escape the recognition by alveolar macrophages, resulting in more effective uptake and drug action. Besides polymeric nanoparticles, other types of nanocarriers, including liposomes and solid lipid nanoparticles, have been used for the pulmonary delivery of protein drugs. A more detailed discussion on these nanocarriers can be found in the following sections.

Inhalable insulin is a powdered form of insulin, delivered with an inhaler into the lungs where it is absorbed. In general, inhaled insulins have been more rapidly absorbed than subcutaneously injected insulin, with a faster peak concentration in serum and more rapid metabolism. Exubera, developed by Inhale Therapeutics (later named Nektar Therapeutics), became the first inhaled insulin product to be marketed in 2006 by Pfizer, but poor sales led Pfizer to withdraw it in 2007. Afrezza, a monomeric inhaled insulin developed by Mannkind, was approved by the FDA in 2014. Dypreza, an inhaled insulin developed by Highlands Pharmaceuticals, was approved for sale in Europe in 2013 and the United States in 2016. The critical issue with inhalable insulin comes from the need to control the dosing accurately; that is not always possible when using a device to administer the drug.

2.4.4 OCULAR

The ocular delivery of proteins is hindered by the blood-retinal barrier and efflux transporters expressed in the posterior segment. The viscosity of formulations also alters ocular drug delivery. High viscosity increases the corneal contact time but leads to reflex tearing and blinking of the eye, which alters the formulations' viscosity.

Ocular delivery is fast growing with at least two products already approved: the anti-vascular endothelial growth factor (anti-VEGF) aptamer and monoclonal antibody (Lucentis and Ranibizumab). Since topically applied conventional dosage forms, such as eye drops, have the main drawbacks of low bioavailability and subsequent low therapeutic efficiency; various new strategies have been developed to overcome the ocular delivery barriers and enhance the bioavailability of proteins via the ocular route of administration. For example, the utilization of chemical chaperones and coadministration of recombinant human hyaluronidase have been attempted to facilitate protein delivery through the ocular route. Since protein aggregation is one of the primary concerns in the formulation of proteins for ocular diseases, a novel strategy to utilize chemical chaperones (protein aggregation inhibitors) was developed to prevent protein misfolding and/or inhibit the self-assembly of aggregation-prone sequences in native protein structures. The coadministration of recombinant hyaluronidases has also been used for decades to increase the penetration of biological drugs across ocular tissue barriers. Hyaluronidases catalyze the degradation of hyaluronic acid, a critical structural component of tissues. Furthermore, various nanocarriers, including polymeric micelles, liposomes, nanospheres, nano wafers, and dendrimers, are being extensively evaluated for their controlled and targeted delivery of proteins via the ocular route. Table 2.3 lists the drugs administered through ocular routes.

Nano wafers are tiny transparent circular or rectangular membranes that contain arrays of drug-loaded nano reservoirs that release drugs in a highly controlled

TABLE 2.3
Ocular Biological Products

Product	Drug	Route	Indications
Cenegermin	Oxervate	Eye drop	Neurotrophic keratitis
Eylea	Aflibercept	Ocular	Wet age-related macular degeneration (WAMD), Diabetic
Lucentis	Ranibizumab	Ocular	macular edema (DME) or Diabetic retinopathy (DR) in DME, Macular edema following retinal vein occlusion (MEtRVO) WAMD, DME or DR in DME, MEtRVO, Myopic choroidal neovascularization (mCNV)

manner and for a longer duration than eye drops (a few hours to several days). They are composed of various polymers such as polyvinyl alcohol, polyvinyl pyrrolidone, hydroxypropyl methylcellulose, and carboxymethyl cellulose. Nano wafers are applied by the patient's fingertip, can withstand constant blinking without removal, release the drug slowly, enhance drug resident time and absorption into ocular tissues, and improve therapeutic efficacy. Furthermore, during drug release, the nano wafer slowly dissolves, rendering ocular surfaces free of polymers.

Drug-loaded contact lenses are also candidates for effective ocular drug delivery and therapy. Contact lenses provide longer drug residence time on the eye, which enhances drug permeation through the cornea. The slow diffusion of drug molecules from the lens matrix offers sustained drug release. The residence time and drug release rate can be further improved by entrapping the drug in nanocarriers and dispersing the drug-loaded nanocarriers in the lens matrix. The application of drug-loaded contact lenses as an ocular delivery system for macromolecules needs to be further explored to achieve the desired therapeutic objectives. However, limitations, including drug leaching during storage and distribution and safety issues related to surface roughness, must be resolved.

2.5 REFERENCE PRODUCT

The reference product must be a product license in the US for FDA submission and EU or US for the EU submission. Attempts are made to remove bridging studies if a non-US product is used as a reference product, if it is approved using essentially the same registration dossier; however, until then, if the goal is to file in the EU and US simultaneously, choosing the US product will be preferred, as approvals can be obtained from the EMA for the reference product.

The reference product may have more than one therapeutic indication. When proposed biological comparability has been demonstrated in one indication, extrapolation of clinical data to other indications of the reference product could be acceptable but needs to be scientifically justified. In case it is unclear whether the safety and efficacy confirmed in one indication would be relevant for another indication, additional data will be required. It is expected that the safety and efficacy can be extrapolated when proposed biological comparability has been demonstrated by thorough physicochemical and structural analyses as well as by in vitro functional tests complemented with clinical data (efficacy and safety and PK/PD data) in one therapeutic indication. Additional data are required in certain situations such as,

- The active substance of the reference product interacts with several receptors that may have a different impact on the tested and non-tested therapeutic indications.
- The active substance itself has more than one active site, and the sites may have a different impact on different therapeutic indications.
- The studied therapeutic indication is not relevant for the others in terms of efficacy or safety, i.e., it is not sensitive to differences in all relevant aspects of efficacy and safety.

3 Development Master Plan

3.1 INTRODUCTION

Companies often begin developing relationships with the wholesaler 18–24 months before the product's market launch to determine the best strategies for commercialization and the appropriate channels for distribution. There are two distribution models that can be adapted. Specialty distribution refers to specialty products or biosimilars that are used to treat chronic indications; for example, Amjevita (adalimumab-atto), a biosimilar developed for the treatment of psoriasis and is typically distributed through a specialty distributor to physician-owned clinics, hospitals, or hospital-owned outpatient clinics. In these settings, the management purchases and stores the biosimilars through a process known as buy-and-bill, which refers to when a healthcare provider purchases, stores, and then administers the product to a patient and after the patient receives the drug, and any other necessary medical care, the provider submits a claim for reimbursement to a third-party payer.

Furthermore, in the full-line distribution model, a pharmaceutical company or manufacturer sells the whole line of its product through a wholesaler. Most of the products are supplied to pharmacies (retail, independent, mail-order) and possibly also physician clinics and hospitals. In some instances, companies may distribute their products via specialty distribution in addition to full-line wholesale distribution. Since there are fewer specialty distributors, hospitals and clinics may face greater expenses during the product-acquiring process using this method, making the full-line model more accessible and affordable. For example, Zirabev (biosimilar of Avastin; used for cancer treatment) is primarily distributed through the specialty model, but it can be distributed through the full-line model for economic reasons.

The best model may vary based on the biosimilar's distribution, cost, and/or product itself. Developing and manufacturing companies design their distribution and commercialization strategies prioritizing access and affordability for the patients. Another factor considered includes how the company–wholesaler relationship can best deliver treatments to each patient, which often requires an understanding of the competitive market in which the biosimilar will compete and how the original biologic's product is being distributed.

To acquire the cost-normalized value of the biosimilars, a series of economic evaluations and comparisons may be required to perform for each product and even for each indication (proposed or licensed), such as cost-effective analysis, cost-benefit analysis, cost-utility analysis, and cost-minimization analysis, with the major focus on the cost control of a marketed product, the total cost of each indication, the average cost per prescription or patient, cost per life-year gained, quality-adjusted life-year gained, quality-of-life-adjusted life expectancy, the number of the severe

DOI: 10.1201/9781003404637-3

adverse medical events avoided, and the number of deaths averted. Clearly, these cost-related analyses would help further improve drug development and utilization, making manufacturing more cost-effective and thus benefiting patients the most.

While it is plausible for the developers to seek out the largest revenue products, such as adalimumab, the most valuable opportunities reside in the products that have not been popular. However, the frequency of approvals is not proportional to the market of the product; nine filgrastim products with total global sales of about $1B compared to four bevacizumab with total sales of more than $10B compared to adalimumab with a market approaching $20B leaves much to discuss. Notably, only one monoclonal antibody, trastuzumab, is included in the WHO list of essential drugs.

In 2021, the regulatory agencies began focusing on decreasing anti-competitive behavior in the biosimilars space, lowering biologic drug prices, and providing further guidance to clarify the regulatory pathway for biosimilars.

- "Anti-competitive practices, such as making false or misleading statements comparing biological reference products and biosimilars, may be slowing progress and hampering the uptake of these important therapies," the FDA, and the Federal Trade Commission (FTC) stated in a joint statement in February 2020. The agencies agreed to take appropriate steps to deter anti-competitive behavior.
- In a news release dated July 20, 2021, the FDA stated that Amgen is making false claims regarding its Neulasta medicine being more effective in its new delivery system Onpro.
- President Biden signed an executive order titled "Promoting Competition in the American Economy," which directs the FTC to issue rules to prevent "unfair anticompetitive conduct or agreements in the prescription drug industries, such as agreements to delay the market entry of generic drugs or biosimilars." The Order also directs the FDA to address a number of issues affecting biosimilars, including: (i) "improving and clarifying interchangeability standards for biological products"; (ii) "supporting biosimilar product adoption by providing effective educational materials and communications to improve understanding of biosimilar and interchangeable products among healthcare providers, patients, and caregivers"; and (iii) "facilitating the development and approval of biosimilar and interchangeable products among healthcare providers, patients, and caregivers."
- A new law, "Advancing Education on Biosimilars Act," now calls for the government to provide educational materials to healthcare providers, patients, and the public to increase awareness, knowledge, and confidence in the safety and efficacy of approved biosimilars.
- The "Star Rating for Biosimilars Act" adds a qualification system to Medicare plans.
- The "Bolstering Innovative Options to Save Immediately on Medicines" (BIOSIM) Act intends to lower biologic drug prices by temporarily increasing reimbursement to ASP plus 8% (from ASP + 6% previously) for providers that employ a biosimilar that is less expensive than the reference product.

- The "Preserve Access to Affordable Generics and Biosimilars Act" changes the FTC Act to presumptively render anticompetitive "pay-for-delay" (also known as "reverse-payment") settlement agreements that prohibit or delay the introduction of generic pharmaceuticals or biosimilars illegal.
- The Inflation Reduction Act (2022) allowed the CMS to reduce the price of biological drugs that had enjoyed a monopoly for more than 12 years unless there is a biosimilar available or its arrival imminent. This was one of the strongest incentives for the entry of new biosimilars.
- The "Pharmacy Benefit Manager Transparency Act of 2023." This bill generally prohibits pharmacy benefit managers (PBMs) from engaging in certain practices when managing prescription drug benefits under a health insurance plan, including charging the plan a different amount than the PBM reimburses the pharmacy. The bill also prohibits PBMs from arbitrarily, unfairly, or deceptively (i) clawing back reimbursement payments or (ii) increasing fees or lowering reimbursements to pharmacies to offset changes to federally funded health plans. PBMs are not subject to these prohibitions if they (i) pass along 100% of any price concession or discount to the health plan and (ii) disclose specified costs, prices, reimbursements, fees, markups, discounts, and aggregate payments received with respect to their PBM services. Further, PBMs must report annually to the FTC certain information about payments received from health plans and fees charged to pharmacies. The FTC and state attorneys general are authorized to enforce the provisions of the bill.
- The "Biosimilar Red Tape Elimination Act" in the Senate suggests removing the interchangeable status of biosimilars as a redundant exercise that reduces the competition and increases the cost to developers.
- Currently, there are 229 bills in the Senate that affect the approval, pricing, distribution, reimbursement, and adoption of biosimilars (www.congress.gov).

3.2 CREATING A PLAN

Enabling a lower-cost alternative to an expensive biological product, biologicals play a significant role. Being a new genre of products, proposed biological development has been marred with many conflicts of understanding that we wish to clear in a description based on our hands-on experience in developing biologicals at the lowest possible cost.

At first, every proposed biological developer must create a detailed and comprehensive Development Master Plan as described below.

Most proposed biological developers face a dilemma in choosing the product to develop because of cost and time constraints for taking the product through regulatory approval. The traditional business development teams follow complex rules of the market, competitors, now and by the time the product is approved, and the cost of goods to decide which product to manufacture. While these considerations have survived the test of time, there are many reasons why these do not always apply to selecting a proposed biological product to develop.

First, unlike chemical generics, competitors' fields will always be much smaller, not for financial reasons but for the need for deep science that is not

Frequency of Approval

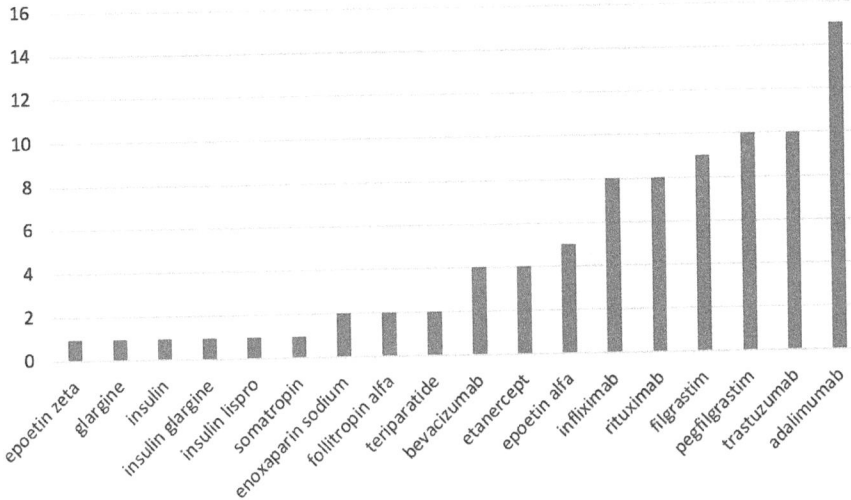

FIGURE 3.1 Frequency of approval of biologicals in the US and EU, as of May 2020 (based on the definition of a proposed biological in each jurisdiction).

available to many. So, regardless of the nature of the product, the competition will always be limited.

Given that almost every proposed biological product can be a blockbuster, a different type of projection is required to qualify a product regardless of the competitors. Figure 3.1 shows the frequency of approval of biologicals in the US and EU.

The developers' common practice is to examine the public domain data, particularly the Biologicals License Application (BLA) documents available [https://www.accessdata.fda.gov/scripts/cder/daf/]. A detailed analysis of the regulatory submissions that led to these products' approval shows high diversity, frequent redundancy, and reliance on studies that may not assure biologicals' safety and efficacy. The paradigm of stepwise development and evaluation suggested by the FDA has also not worked. We have sufficient data to indicate that a significant change in the biological approval guidance is required to remove redundant testing and reduce the risk of approval of unsafe biologicals.

Table 3.1 lists over 1100 analytical similarities, 96 animal pharmacology, 42 in vitro/ex vitro pharmacology, 52 clinical pharmacology, and 32 clinical efficacy studies. Here are the highlights of the compiled data:

- The FDA did not review 27 animal pharmacology studies, labeling them redundant or unnecessary.
- No animal pharmacology or in vitro/ex-vitro study failed.
- A few clinical pharmacology studies had to be repeated to meet acceptance criteria due to the wrong choice of the study population. None failed.
- No clinical efficacy studies failed where the primary endpoints did not meet, post hoc analysis, and additional scientific justification. In two cases, higher

TABLE 3.1
Studies Submitted for Licensing of Biologicals Approved by the FDA

Licensed Product	Analytical	Animal Pharmacology	In Vitro/Ex-vitro Pharmacology	Clinical Pharmacology	Clinical Efficacy	Total
Humira						
Adalimumab-atto	41	2	0	1	2	46
adalimumab-adaz	52	5	1	4	1	63
Adalimumab-adbm	70	6 (2)	26 (10)	2	1	105
adalimumab-afzb	25	1	0	3	2	31
adalimumab-bwwd	38	2	0	2	2	44
Avastin						
bevacizumab-awwb	56	7 (2)	0	1	1	65
bevacizumab-bvzr	42	2	4	1	1	50
Epogen						
epoetin alfa-epbx	32	15 (13)	0	4	0	79
Enbrel						
etanercept-szzs	53	5	0	4	1	88
etanercept-ykro	52	3	0	1	1	57
Neupogen						
filgrastim-aafi	38	1	0	3	0	42
filgrastim-sndz	41	5	0	5	1	52
infliximab-abda	52	3	0	1	1	57
Remicade						
infliximab-axxq	61	1	2	1	1	66
infliximab-dyyb	33	4 (2)	2	4	5	48
infliximab-qbtx	51	2	0	2	1	80
Neulasta						
pegfilgrastim-bmez	NA	13 (8)	0	2	2	17
pegfilgrastim-cbqv	31	1	2	2	0	36
pegfilgrastim-jmdb	31	2	0	2	1	36
Rituxan						
rituximab-abbs	50	1	1	1	1	171
rituximab-pvvr	40	2	0	1	2	98
Herceptin						
trastuzumab-anns	27	5	2	1	1	111
trastuzumab-dkst	37	2	2	1	1	84
trastuzumab-dttb	48	2	0	1	1	99
trastuzumab-pkrb	44	2	0	1	1	48
trastuzumab-qyyp	44	2	0	1	1	48

immunogenicity was overcome by minor manufacturing process changes. No product was rejected based on a failed efficacy study.

- There was no correlation between submissions for the same molecule; trastuzumab had 48–111 total studies by different developers.

In summary, all analytical similarity testing met the acceptance criteria, the animal pharmacology studies added little to the knowledge, all clinical pharmacology studies reached the criteria, and even when there was a difference in clinical efficacy studies, these were overcome by discussing data and allowing marketing authorization. Given these observations, a proposed biological the developers have an opportunity to present to FDA testing protocols that may not be as extensive as those used to approve all current products.

The analysis presented in Table 3.1 is for the developers to meet with the FDA, first in a Biologicals Advisory Meeting that requires expressing the biological entity at a small scale with initial analytical similarity testing. This meeting should be followed by Type 2 meetings to secure an agreement with the FDA on the minimal studies required.

3.3 INTELLECTUAL PROPERTY

Given that it will take 3–4 years to get to a regulatory filing if you start a project today, the total number of choices available to you is well over 100; why not choose a product with the following attributes, making the following metrics highly valuable? (Table 6.4)

- Less Complex Structure: fewer analytical tests are required; a product with fewer PTMs is less complicated.
- Easier to Express: less batch-to-batch variability; a fusion protein or Mab is more difficult
- Has an established market known for its safety and efficacy, reducing redundant testing; molecules such as hormones and cytokines are here to stay forever; MAbs will change with time?
- Does not require large CAPEX: MAbs will take many times more CAPEX than cytokines
- Has already been approved as a proposed biological in the EU or USA: being number two or three is an advantage to many (Table 3.2).

3.3.1 COGs

The COGs can be controlled: most products will cost the same within a small variation if you follow the development cycle to reduce your future COGs. The cost of goods is often considered a selection criterion, but this is a poor indicator since biological drug production costs are relatively uniform, such as $150–$300/g from monoclonal antibodies; cytokines vary not that much in their category. Most of the cost goes into the media cost since production produces a carbon-based entity.

TABLE 3.2

Patent Expiry (Date) of Biological Products Licensed by the FDA

Albumin (human) (1990-11-16)

Collagenase (2004-01-16)

Hyaluronidase (2004-02-24)

Urokinase (2004-02-24)

Fibrinogen (human) (2004-02-27)

Aprotinin (2004-03-17)

Insulin human (2004-03-24)

Interferon beta-1b (2004-03-28)

Immunoglobulin g (2004-04-21)

Parathyroid hormone (2004-04-21)

Dermatophagoides farinae (2004-07-21)

Dermatophagoides pteronyssinus (2004-07-21)

Anti-inhibitor coagulant complex (2004-08-18)

Histamine phosphate (2004-11-10)

Interferon alfa-2b (2004-12-28)

Plasma protein fraction (human) (2005-01-19)

Natalizumab (2005-01-30)

Asparaginase (2005-03-08)

Filgrastim (2005-08-23)

Factor IX complex (2005-10-25)

Tuberculin purified protein derivative (2006-03-06)

Rho (d) immune globulin (2006-11-25)

Gonadotropin, chorionic (2007-01-30)

Sebelipase alfa (2007-04-17)

Human immunoglobulin g (2007-07-31)

Antithrombin iii (human) (2008-07-25)

Immune globulin (human) (2008-09-24)

Anakinra (2008-12-24)

Alemtuzumab (2010-05-11)

Abciximab (2010-09-14)

Interferon alfa-n3   (2011-03-01)

Bacillus calmette-guerin (2011-05-03)

Antihemophilic factor/von willebrand factor complex (human) (2011-07-19)

Pancrelipase (amylase lipase protease) (2012-01-16)

Aldesleukin (2012-02-03)

Etanercept (2012-03-07)

Epoetin alfa (2012-08-15)

Thrombin human (2012-09-09)

Becaplermin (2012-10-10)

Ibritumomab tiuxetan (2012-11-13)

Pegfilgrastim (2013-12-03)

Bevacizumab (2014-01-25)

Reslizumab (2014-06-17)

(Continued)

TABLE 3.2 (*Continued*)
Patent Expiry (Date) of Biological Products Licensed by the FDA

Cetuximab (2014-08-10)

Trastuzumab (2014-08-10)

Trastuzumab

Hyaluronidase-oysk (2014-08-10)

Pegaspargase (2014-10-20)

Von willebrand factor (recombinant) (2014-11-14)

Denileukin diftitox (2015-02-01)

Rituximab (2015-02-01)

Hyaluronidase (human recombinant) (2015-02-01)

Sargramostim (2015-02-01)

Imiglucerase (2015-03-24)

Menotropins (fsh lh) (2015-09-29)

Palifermin (2015-09-29)

Urofollitropin (2015-09-29)

Peginterferon alfa-2b (2015-11-02)

Basiliximab (2016-05-16)

Daclizumab (2016-05-16)

Latrodectus mactans (2016-05-18)

Alteplase (2016-05-22)

Equine thymocyte immune globulin (2016-09-05)

Ambrosia artemisiifolia (2016-11-26)

Denosumab (2016-12-23)

Insulin lispro (2017-01-10)

Infliximab (2017-04-04)

Panitumumab (2017-05-05)

Adalimumab (2017-09-26)

Reteplase (2017-09-26)

Blinatumomab (2018-04-21)

Insulin aspart (2018-05-19)

Rilonacept (2018-09-25)

Romiplostim (2018-10-23)

Human plasma proteins (2018-12-10)

Interferon beta-1a (2020-01-14)

Interferon gamma-1b (2020-01-14)

Palivizumab (2020-05-03)

Capromab pendetide (2020-08-21)

Ranibizumab (2020-08-24)

Gemtuzumab ozogamicin (2020-11-28)

Ocriplasmin (2020-12-21)

Abatacept (2021-02-15)

Golimumab (2021-03-07)

Rasburicase (2021-05-01)

Dornase alfa (2021-09-04)

(*Continued*)

TABLE 3.2 (*Continued*)
Patent Expiry (Date) of Biological Products Licensed by the FDA

Tenecteplase (2021-10-30)
Insulin detemir (2021-11-19)
Laronidase (2021-11-30)
Follitropin alfa/beta (2022-01-22)
Pertuzumab (2022-05-17)
Peginterferon alfa-2a (2022-08-01)
Corticorelin ovine triflutate (2022-08-05)
Omalizumab (2022-08-14)
Darbepoetin alfa (2022-08-29)
Pegvisomant (2023-01-09)
Imciromab pentetate (2023-03-05)
Thyrotropin alfa (2023-06-24)
Agalsidase beta (2023-10-01)
Selumetinib (2023-12-12)
Albiglutide (2025-01-04)
Antihemophilic factor (human) (2025-01-04)
Insulin aspart recombinant (2025-01-04)
Lixisenatide (2025-01-04)
Methoxide polyethylene glycol-epoetin beta (2025-01-04)
Aflibercept (2025-03-15)
Ramucirumab (2025-03-15)
Belimumab (2025-05-20)
Insulin glulisine recombinant (2025-05-23)
Certolizumab pegol (2025-11-08)
Ipilimumab (2025-11-08)
Fremanezumab-vfrm (2025-11-14)
Calfactant (2026-01-10)
Tocilizumab (2026-04-13)
Eculizumab (2026-04-27)
Inotuzumab ozogamicin (2026-06-23)
Mepolizumab (2026-06-23)
Ocrelizumab (2026-06-23)
Ofatumumab (2026-06-23)
Raxibacumab (2026-06-23)
Coagulation factor ix (recombinant) (2026-07-13)
Desirudin recombinant (2026-08-02)
Poractant alfa (2026-11-02)
Benralizumab (2027-01-11)
Galsulfase (2027-06-13)
Evolocumab (2027-08-23)
Ustekinumab (2027-11-30)
Capmatinib (2027-12-12)
Human fibrinogen, human thrombin (2028-05-22)

(Continued)

TABLE 3.2 (*Continued*)
Patent Expiry (Date) of Biological Products Licensed by the FDA

Mecasermin rinfabate recombinant (2028-06-19)
Ado-trastuzumab emtansine (2028-10-22)
Belatacept (2028-12-05)
Osilodrostat (2029-03)
Opicapone (2029-12-12)
Ozanimod (2029-12-12)
Canakinumab (2030-03-29)
Abobotulinumtoxina (2030-03-30)
Asparaginase erwinia chrysanthemi (2030-03-30)
Incobotulinumtoxina (2030-03-30)
Dulaglutide (2030-05-05)
Metreleptin (2030-05-05)
Brentuximab vedotin (2030-05-26)
Insulin degludec (2030-06-24)
Sipuleucel-t (2030-07-19)
Necitumumab (2030-09-08)
Brodalumab (2030-10-08)
Secukinumab (2030-10-08)
Nivolumab (2031-02-04)
Pembrolizumab (2031-02-04)
Insulin detemir recombinant (2031-04-01)
Vedolizumab (2031-05-02)
Idursulfase (2031-06-08)
Ecallantide (2031-06-10)
Human c1-esterase inhibitor (2031-06-10)
Elotuzumab (2031-08-05)
Olaratumab (2031-08-05)
Siltuximab (2031-08-05)
Sarilumab (2031-10-11)
Alirocumab (2031-10-25)
Alirocumab (2031-10-25)
Asfotase alfa (2031-10-25)
Elosulfase alfa (2031-10-25)
Insulin aspart
insulin degludec (2031-10-25)
Insulin degludec
liraglutide (2031-10-25)
Insulin glargine recombinant (2031-10-25)
Insulin lispro recombinant (2031-10-25)
Ixekizumab (2031-10-25)
Obinutuzumab (2031-10-25)
Peginterferon beta-1a (2031-10-25)

(*Continued*)

TABLE 3.2 *(Continued)*
Patent Expiry (Date) of Biological Products Licensed by the FDA

Daratumumab (2031-10-28)
Somatropin (2031-12-05)
Eptinezumab-jjmr (2031-12-12)
Selpercatinib (2031-12-12)
Selpercatinib (2031-12-12)
Atezolizumab (2032-08-13)
Avelumab (2032-08-14)
Durvalumab (2032-08-14)
Talimogene laherparepvec (2032-08-30)
Ziv-aflibercept (2032-10-31)
Ripretinib (2032-12-12)
2033–2039
Choriogonadotropin alfa (2033-02-06)
Alglucosidase alfa (2033-03-11)
Insulin recombinant human insulin susp isophane recombinant human (2033-03-11)
Sacrosidase (2033-03-11)
Dupilumab (2033-03-14)
Coagulation factor viia (recombinant) (2033-04-24)
Bezlotoxumab (2033-09-09)
Pemigatinib (2033-12-12)
Sacituzumab govitecan-hziy (2033-12-12)
Tucatinib (2033-12-12)
Ravulizumab-cwvz (2034-03-07)
Idarucizumab (2034-07-31)
Dinutuximab (2034-10-06)
Guselkumab (2035-02-24)
Obiltoxaximab (2035-02-24)
Isatuximab-irfc (2035-10-05)
Taliglucerase alfa (2036-02-11)
Velaglucerase alfa (2036-02-11)
Polatuzumab vedotin-piiq (2039-10-22).

Only the carbon in and carbon out formula always works. More details are provided below in the selection of the manufacturing process.

3.3.2 EXTRAPOLATION AND SUBSTITUTION

A proposed biological product received extrapolation of all indications approved for the reference product as of the date and allowed, barring any intellectual property in the marketing authorization. The developer should provide a justification document to claim extrapolation in light of the observed similarity; there may be situations where the extrapolation may not be allowed because of the peculiarities found

in a proposed biological product. Suppose the reference product receives marketing authorization for additional indications without making any changes to the reference product. In that case, the developers may request a modification to their label claim, regardless of the intellectual property involved, since the developer and the innovator company resolve this issue.

The European Medicines Agency (EMA) does not allow automatic substitution of a proposed biological product for the reference product. However, various jurisdictions within the EU judge; in the US, substitution requires additional testing to demonstrate no more safety risk and no less efficacy upon switching and alternating; the FDA has yet to approve any product with this designation.

3.3.3 STUDY WAIVERS

An application for marketing authorization of a proposed biological product may rely upon the previous determination of the reference product's safety, purity, and potency, including any clinical QT/QTc interval prolongation and proarrhythmic potential and drug–drug interactions. If such studies were not required for the reference product, then these data generally would not be needed for the marketing authorization of a proposed biological product.

A proposed biological product is considered not to have a "new active ingredient," a pediatric assessment is generally not required if such a waiver has been awarded to the reference product. However, where a proposed biological product has a different formulation, the developer should submit a statement asserting why the formulation does not create any additional pediatric use risk.

Specific studies, like carcinogenicity, reproductive toxicity, etc., are not required for biosimilars.

3.3.4 PUBLIC DOMAIN KNOWLEDGE

Collect and analyze all available reports in public, including the EPARs, the BLA Review documents, and similar documents made available by other agencies listed above. When relying upon published scientific literature, the developers must ensure that the publications do not have any conflict of interest, such as a manufacturer publishing its data submitted for marketing authorization with conclusions drawn that may differ from the regulatory authority's decision. While the US FDA makes BLA details available for many new products, the developers may request this information using the Freedom of Information Act provisions on a small fee basis. While these documents are redacted for confidential information, the developer will have sufficient scientific knowledge to use the available information best.

Collect and analyze all available information available on approved biologicals to the reference product selected by the developer. The regulatory information, as enumerated above, is also available for biologicals. In particular, the developers can benefit from prescribing information approved for these products. The developers may also want to create an internal library of all available scientific reports on the reference product, its active ingredient, and the technology employed in the manufacturing and testing of biological products. Some commercial vendors may have already secured and sold this information to companies. Regulatory information should be considered only from the following countries: Western Europe, USA, Japan, Canada, or Australia. Some emerging market regulatory authorities have adopted a chemical-generic approach, allow study waivers, and do not assure safety and efficacy.

3.4 EXPRESSION SYSTEM

Generally, some quality attributes are strictly related to proteins' expression and the cell line's selection. When a new biological product is developed, the selected cell line product is characterized and taken through all three development phases. In biologicals, the cell line must produce a similar product, and that can be challenging if the product has many post-translational modifications, higher molecular weight, and a highly complex structure. In creating monoclonal antibodies, a single cell (monoclonal) is used to develop a uniform cell line, which may not necessarily be the best choice. The developers should first conduct analytical testing of the reference product to establish the quality attributes required before selecting a cell line colony to avoid extensive testing later to justify any analytical differences in the expression of proteins from the fixed cell line. It is essential to understand that a high titer cell line reduces the size of the bioreactor only; for low-dose products like cytokines, the titer differences do not affect the size or cost as much as the suppliers of new cell lines tout it.

3.5 RELEASE SPECIFICATION

When a new biological product is developed, the specification is established based on multiple lots' attributes. There is rarely any question of why a particular specification is used to release a product, notwithstanding known limitations common to the dosage form. When a proposed biological product is developed, the boundaries of the specifications are already drawn to match despite the realization that the expression systems are inevitably different. So are the upstream and downstream processes. It is like walking a fine line to minimize the studies required to prove that any deviations are not clinically meaningful from the reference product posed; biological companies must have a deep understanding of the product, the technology, the testing methodologies, and creative minds to ensure the regulatory agencies that there is no clinically meaningful difference between a proposed biological and the reference product.

Multiple reference products should be used to establish specifications for qualifying drugs and drug products. The number of reference product lots depends on the variability of the quality attributes in the reference product. Generally, there is not likely to be a considerable variation in protein concentration, bioassay, post-translational modifications, impurities, and other physical properties of the reference product since the manufacturer has validated the manufacturing process over time. Since a proposed biological product does not have access to the in-process controls, earlier lots of offered biological products may show higher variation, making it essential to obtain extensive data on the variability of attributes in the reference product lots. The release specifications should include assay, bioassay, physical attributes, subvisible particles, total impurities, individual impurities, aggregates, and post-translational modifications.

3.5.1 REFERENCE STANDARD

Comparing a proposed biological product to a publicly available standard, e.g., a pharmacopeia monograph, or using a reference standard is *not* allowed for comparative testing to establish biosimilarity. It is emphasized that any pharmacopeia monograph specifications or a reference standard provided by third parties are not considered appropriate to demonstrate biosimilarity.

Pharmacopoeia reference standards are not suitable to conduct any comparative study, and their use is limited only to the qualification of test methods. The developer develops a qualified reference standard internally based on its own fully characterized batch.

If a suitable, publicly available, and well-established reference standard exists for the protein, a physicochemical and functional comparison of a proposed biological product with this standard may also provide helpful information. Although studies with such a reference standard may be beneficial, they are insufficient to satisfy the requirement to demonstrate the biosimilarity of a proposed biological product to the reference product. For example, if an international standard for potency calibration is available, a comparison of a proposed biological product's relative potency with this standard should be performed. As recommended in ICH Q6B, an in-house reference standard(s) should always be qualified and used to control the manufacturing process and product.

An in-house reference standard is typically developed from early development lots or lots used in a clinical study. Additional reference standards may be qualified later in development and for submission. Ideally, the developers will have established and properly qualified primary and working reference standards representative of proposed biological product lots used in clinical studies that support the application.

The reference product lot is typically qualified as an initial reference standard to develop a proposed biological product. Once clinical lots of a proposed biological product have been manufactured, it is expected that one of these lots will be properly qualified (including bridging to previous reference standards) for use as a reference standard for release and stability as well as comparative analytical testing. Once an in-house reference standard is properly qualified, there should be sufficient quantities to use throughout the development of a proposed biological product. All reference standards used during the development of a proposed biological product should be properly qualified. In addition to release testing methods, the qualification protocol for reference standards should include all analytical methods that report the result relative to the reference standard.

For all methods where the result is reported relative to the reference standard, the potency assignment of 100% should include a narrow acceptable potency range and ensure control over product drift. For example, the developers should consider using a pre-determined two-sided confidence interval (CI) of the mean of the replicates, where the mean relative potency and the 95% CI are included within a sufficiently narrow range (e.g., 90%–110%). There should be an evaluation across the history of multiple reference standard qualifications to address potential drift.

The developers should not use a correction factor to account for differences in, for example, potency or biological activity between reference standards.

Using reference standards inadequately qualified for analytical methods that report results relative to the reference standard will likely raise concerns regarding the comparative analytical assessment. If applicable, one approach to address these concerns may be to store the reference product lots under conditions that maintain stability long term, if feasible. Before applying, the prospective developer should re-evaluate a proposed biological product and the reference product lots using the same reference standard for those methods that report the result relative to the reference standard.

3.5.2 Analytical Assessment

Analytical assessment comprises physicochemical and functional properties and forms the backbone for establishing biosimilarity. How much a biosimilar candidate matches the reference product shall remain a debate because reference products are approved based on whatever quality attributes they present; a biosimilar must check these, even though the attributes of the reference product may not be ideal. An analytical assessment begins with understanding the variability of quality attributes of the reference product, but not all attributes need to be studied side by side.

The following non-legacy attributes are related to the product and, therefore, require a side-by-side comparison with the reference product:

- Amino Acid Sequence, Primary Structure: Peptide mapping (LC-MS), Peptide mass fingerprint (MALDI-MS), MALDI Time of flight mass spectrometry (TOF), and MS amino acid sequencing.
- Higher-Order Structure, Conformation: Fluorescence, Far and near Ultraviolet (UV) CD, Differential scanning calorimetry (DSC), Nuclear Magnetic Resonance (NMR), Nuclear Magnetic Resonance (SPR), and Enzyme Linked Immunosorbent Assay (ELISA).
- Binding: Cell-based assays, SPR, ELISA, and other methods are available.
- Degradation Profile: molecular structure integrity is based on structure; the forced and shelf-life stability should demonstrate a similar profile.
- Impurity Profile: impurities may have lesser potency, but an unmatched impurity is an immunogenicity risk.
- Aggregates
- Physical Properties: since biosimilars can have different formulations, physical property variability is based on testing multiple batches of the biosimilar candidate. Release specification should include surfactant range if used.

The legacy attributes are established without the need for side-by-side testing:

- Protein Content: ±3% variation or higher is supported by data from the reference product
- Potency: ±15% variation or higher is supported by data from the reference product.
- Impurities: NMT 3% or higher is supported by data from the reference product.
- Compendial standards of subvisible particles, residual DNA, fill volume, and sterility.

The testing methods must be suitable, not necessarily validated for side-by-side testing, since this testing design overcomes any method accuracy issues.

Since analytical assessment is the core of establishing biosimilarity, issues like non-compliance with CFR 21 Part 11, data integrity, and sample collection and recording are the typical findings in the Complete Response Letters issued by the FDA to biosimilar developers.

3.6 NONCLINICAL TESTING

The use of nonhuman primates, the only species with relevant receptors, is often recommended to conduct PK studies in a small number of animals, particularly for monoclonal antibodies. However, while these studies may provide additional support to structural similarity, they cannot be of any value in justifying differences in the analytical assessment.

Regulatory agencies are now suggesting avoiding animal testing of even new biological even if an animal species can show a response, except if the carcinogenicity potential exists. In addition, the FDA/CDER now also encourages exploring the use of New Approach Methodologies to improve regulatory efficiency and potentially expedite new drug development in line with the European Union legislation on the protection of animals used for scientific purposes.

Alternative approaches to animal testing models are based on human and animal cells, organoids, organ-on-chips, and in silico modeling, providing opportunities to develop better and more predictive scientific tools to protect human and animal health and the environment. One trend of the last 10 years has seen nonclinical in vivo testing replaced by in vitro assays to reflect changes in animal protection legislation.

Animal toxicology studies are no longer required, removed in the FDA Modernization Act 2.0, and the term is replaced with "non-clinical," which is defined as follows: "cell-based assays, organ chips and micro-physiological systems, sophisticated computer modeling, other human biology-based test methods, and animal tests." However, many agencies, particularly in developing countries, continue to require multi-dose animal toxicology testing that is entirely useless.

Once a product has been scaled to a development level, the developers may consider conducting nonclinical pharmacology studies where needed. Agencies encourage the

TABLE 3.3

Common Critical Quality Attributes

Quality Attribute	Criticality	Potential Impact	Suggested Analytical Methods
Amino acid sequence	Very High	Efficacy, Safety	Peptide Mapping, MS, Edelman Degradation
Glycan structure and content	Very High	Efficacy, Safety	Glycan Analysis
Biological Activity	Very High	Efficacy, Safety	Bioassay
Immunochemical Identity	Very High	Efficacy, Safety	SDS PAGE+ immunoblotting, Immunoassay
High Order Structure	High	Efficacy, Safety	Spectrophotometric and thermodynamic Methods
Isoform Distribution	High	Efficacy	Isoelectric Focusing
Insoluble Aggregates	High	Safety	Light Obscuration
High Molecular Weight Aggregates	High	Safety	SE HPLC, AUC, SDS PAGE
Protein Content	High	Efficacy	UV; use HPLC as an orthogonal method
Host Cell Proteins	High	Safety	SPR, Cell-Based Assay
Receptor Binding	High	Efficacy	SPR, Cell-based Assay
Truncated Forms	Low	Efficacy	reference product HPLC, other Chromatography
Deamidation, Oxidation	Low	Efficacy	Chromatography

developers to justify waivers for conducting nonclinical studies based on the analytical assessment conducted, prior public knowledge about the product's toxicity, and the relevance of animal data to the safety and efficacy of the product. Recently, the agencies have begun to accept waivers even for complex molecules. The developers should understand that the purpose of animal PK studies is to remove any structural similarity since the disposition characteristics of the product may indicate differences in the structure and any immunogenic response that might affect clearance from the body (Table 3.3).

3.7   CLINICAL PHARMACOLOGY ASSESSMENT

The developers should realize that if a PK/pharmacodynamic (PD) study has failed and any residual uncertainty related to the failure is not resolved, then clinical safety and efficacy will not be allowed by the agencies to provide additional proof of biosimilarity, regardless of the size of the clinical efficacy study proposed by the developers.

However, where an efficacy study is conducted, its design must include justification of the indicators chosen to test the product where multiple indications are allowed through extrapolation. The study size should first present the effect size analysis (M1) based on public domain data. An equivalence interval (M2) was decided based on clinical judgment and a rational argument justifying the M2 value.

The choice of study model, equivalence margin vs. non-inferiority, should be explained. A critical element of these studies is the population demographic, which is often difficult to make a practical choice, particularly in anticancer drugs. While naïve patients' option is always desirable, achieving these criteria is often impossible. These complications of safety and efficacy studies make them less reliable than the PK/PD/Immunogenicity testing. When conducted, the developers are encouraged to use clinical markers rather than hard efficacy results where possible, realizing that the study's purpose is not to demonstrate that a proposed biological product is effective. Still, it is equally effective when compared to the reference product. Clinical markers that are relatively easier to evaluate provide greater robustness to the study than the hard efficacy results. Finally, a safety and efficacy study aims to remove any remaining residual uncertainty and not provide proof of biosimilarity based on the study results alone.

The PK/PD studies are pivotal to establishing analytical similarity, in some instances, immunogenicity similarity and, where applicable, bioavailability. Generally, studies in healthy subjects will be more meaningful for two reasons: first, to recruit subjects with a narrow demographic to reduce inter and intra-subject variability. Second, to minimize the impact of disease and related treatments on the disposition profile. However, in some instances where the likelihood of anti-drug antibody (ADA) production is very high, particularly for an endogenous-related product, exposing it to healthy subjects requiring a patient population may be unethical. Regardless of the choice of the population, the goal should be to reduce the number of subjects in the study; one approach that the developers may take is to conduct a two-arm (two doses) parallel two-phase (dose 1, dose 2) study with a follow-up suitable for immunogenicity evaluation; there may be situations where PD determination may restrict the use of this model. The developers may also conduct a post hoc analysis should a study fail to meet the predetermined acceptance criteria to enable a discussion of whether the pre-determined criteria could have been made broader. The purpose of the post hoc analysis is not to change the acceptance criteria retroactively but to determine if the failed study constitutes a significant residual uncertainty. Post hoc analysis may not include additional characterization of results closer to the middle of the acceptance range, as erroneously suggested in some guidelines by other agencies.

Clinical pharmacology comprises studies about what the body does to the drug (PK) and what the drug does to the body (PD), profiling of which *often* cannot be adequately predicted from analytical assessment, functional assays, and nonclinical studies alone, unlike generic chemical drugs where chemical equivalence is established. Given the complexity of the molecular structure, clinical pharmacology studies are used to ascertain further any differences in the molecule's structure that may impact the safety and efficacy of the product.

It is essential to comprehend how immunogenic proteins are to create biologics and vaccines. Increased immunogenicity can result in decreased effectiveness or unfavorable immunological responses, such as allergic reactions or the production of neutralizing antibodies. All proteins are immunogenic; it is a fact. The acquired or antigen-specific immune response involves T and B lymphocytes (T and B Cells). If the immunogenicity profile differs but cannot impact the disposition profile, the differences will be meaningless and unnecessary to compare, as in the case of insulins. During the PK trial, data on immunogenicity and safety should be gathered. Some options include ADA production rate, kinetics, and assessment of their impact on PK (and PD) using a predetermined group study of ADA-negative and ADA-positive participants. In vitro, immunogenicity assays might improve the functional, analytical assessment even if they wouldn't replace the immunogenicity assessment in the PK study. Short-term immunogenicity analyses' findings might not correspond to the actual usage of biologics, especially biosimilars. Due to the small population exposed and the greater scrutiny of patient care in the clinical trial setting, rare ADA-related side events might not be identified in the premarketing phase. Therefore, it is advised that risk management and pharmacovigilance strategies that include monitoring other adverse medication events monitor immunogenicity.

One argument widely presented to test biosimilars in patients is to ensure the safety of immune responses in patients. Here, the understanding about therapeutic proteins is widely misunderstood. Antigens from the extracellular space and sometimes also endogenous ones are enclosed into endocytic vesicles and presented on the cell surface by Major Histocompatibility Complex class II (MHC II) molecules to the helper T cells expressing CD4 molecule. Only antigen presentation cells (APCs) such as dendritic cells (DCs), B cells, or macrophages express MHC-II molecules on their surface in substantial quantity, so the expression of MHC-II molecules is more cell-specific than MHC-I. These fragments are then presented on the surface of cells by MHC II molecules, a process crucial for immune system recognition and response. However, the interaction between these peptides and the immune system can vary depending on an individual's genetic background, particularly the alleles of MHC II they possess. This genetic variation influences the array of peptides that MHC II can present.

The developers should realize that the purpose of clinical studies is *not* to characterize the product (already done in the development of RP) but to *compare* a proposed biological product with the reference product. This premise requires a different approach.

As a matter of clarification, the developers are advised that a classic "phase 1" study is a standalone study to characterize a new drug's disposition characteristics. A classic "phase 3" study is a placebo-controlled study to establish safety and efficacy; neither of these applies to biologicals—as a result, the use of the "phase" terminology should be avoided. The correct terminology is comparative clinical pharmacology and comparative efficacy testing.

Clinical pharmacology studies are an extension of the analytical assessment, a biological tool to identify the structural difference that is impossible to study by any other testing method.

3.7.1 SCOPE OF STUDIES

As a scientific matter, agencies expect the developers to conduct comparative human PK (if the route of administration allows such study to be meaningful) and PD studies (if there is a relevant PD measure(s)) and a clinical immunogenicity assessment, where required to remove any residual uncertainty about the safety and efficacy of a proposed biological product after the completion of all prior studies in a stepwise manner. In certain cases, the results of clinical pharmacology studies, as shown below, may provide adequate data to support the conclusion that there is no clinically meaningful difference between a proposed biological product and the reference product to allow marketing authorization of a proposed biological product. [If a route administers a biological product without a definable blood concentration profile, the developers may justify waiving PK studies. Less complex biological products that are well-characterized and where it is established that variations in immunogenicity do not affect clinical efficacy, the developers may justify a waiver of clinical immunogenicity studies, particularly in the case of insulin products.]

- A human PK study demonstrating similar exposure (e.g., serum concentration over time) for a proposed biological product and the reference product may support a demonstration of biosimilarity.
- A human PD study demonstrating a similar effect on a relevant PD measure(s) related to effectiveness or specific safety concerns (except for immunogenicity, evaluated separately) represents even more robust support for a biosimilarity determination. Even if relevant PD measures are unavailable, sensitive PD endpoints may be assessed if such an assessment reduces uncertainty about biosimilarity. The PK and PD studies may be combined.

Notably, the PK and PD parameters are generally more sensitive than clinical efficacy endpoints in assessing the similarity of a proposed biological product and the reference product. For example, an effect on thyroid-stimulating hormone levels would provide a more sensitive comparison of two thyroxine products than an effect on clinical symptoms of `. The same holds for evaluating filgrastim and erythropoietin products, where the endpoints of change in white and red blood cells serve as a more objective tool to assess these products' efficacy.

Even in those cases where there remains residual uncertainty about biosimilarity, the data from PK and PD studies provide a scientific basis for a selective and targeted approach to subsequent comparative safety and efficacy testing.

3.7.2 Study Plan

Comparative human PK and PD studies should use a population, dose(s), and route of administration (where the option is available) that are adequately sensitive to detect differences in PK and PD profiles. However, one significant difference exists between evaluating a proposed biological product and a stand-alone biological product. The purpose of the assessment of a proposed biological product involves a comparative evaluation, not a characterization of the PK/PD profiles; as a result, the developers may choose a population that is least likely to provide highly variable results to minimize the population size, as well as to enhance the ability of the study to differentiate a proposed biological product and the reference product. This concept is different from the considerations when developing a new product.

The developer should provide a scientific justification for the selection of the human PK and PD study population (e.g., patients versus healthy subjects) and parameters, taking into consideration the relevance and sensitivity of such population and parameters, the population and parameters studied for the marketing authorization for the reference product, as well as the current knowledge of the intra-subject and inter-subject variability of human PK and PD for the reference product.

It is recommended that the developer consider the time it takes for a PD measure to change and the possibility of nonlinear PK in designing study protocols.

Agencies also encourage consideration of the role of modeling and simulation in designing comparative human PK and PD studies. *In silico* modeling of PK/PD studies is a powerful tool to prevent the need for clinical efficacy studies.

The design of a PK study depends on various factors, including clinical context, safety, and PK characteristics of the reference product (target-mediated disposition, linear or non-linear PK, time-dependency, half-life, etc.) Furthermore, bioanalytical assays should be appropriate for their intended use and adequately validated.

- Healthy Subject vs. Patient: Clinical PK and PD studies should be conducted in healthy subjects if the product can be safely administered. A study in healthy subjects is considered more sensitive in evaluating the product similarity because it is likely to produce less PK and PD variability compared with a study in patients with potential confounding factors such as underlying and concomitant disease and concomitant medications. If safety or ethical considerations preclude the participation of healthy subjects in human PK and PD studies for certain products (e.g., immunogenicity or known toxicity from the RP) or if PD biomarkers can only be relevant in patients with the relevant condition or disease, the clinical pharmacology studies should be conducted in such patients. A population that is representative of the patient population to which the drug is targeted will be desirable but not required if the selected population is capable of demonstrating the potential difference between a proposed biological product and the reference product
- Study Size: The total number of subjects studied should provide adequate statistical power for PK and, when relevant, PD similarity assessment. Data analysis should be conducted according to the pre-specified analysis plan and any post hoc statistical analysis is only exploratory. The developers should realize that the purpose of the PK/PD studies is to compare, not characterize, the PK/PD profiles; given the scientific argument that both studies will provide a better assessment of the structural variations, a highly selected population to reduce intra- and inter-subject variability may be more suitable. In the past, several failed PK studies required retesting in a restricted population, such as subjects with a narrow range of BMI, age, gender, and race, to demonstrate biosimilarity.
- Study Design: To evaluate clinical PK and PD similarity for developing proposed biological products, two study designs are particularly relevant: crossover and parallel.
    - Crossover Design: A single-dose, randomized crossover study is generally preferred for PK similarity assessments. A crossover study is

recommended for a product with a short half-life (e.g., shorter than 5 days), a rapid PD response (e.g., the time of onset, maximal effect, and disappearance in conjunction with drug exposure), and a low anticipated incidence of immunogenicity. This design is considered the most sensitive to assess PK similarity and can provide reliable estimates of differences in exposure with a minimum number of subjects. A multiple-dose design may be appropriate for PD similarity assessments when the PD effect is delayed or otherwise not parallel to the single-dose drug PK profile. The course of appearance and disappearance of immunogenicity and its relation to the washout period should be considered for studies using a crossover design.

- Parallel Design: Many biological products have a long half-life and elicit immunogenic responses. A parallel-group design is appropriate for products with a long half-life or for products where repeated exposures can lead to an increased immune response affecting the PK and PD similarity assessments. This design is also appropriate for diseases that exhibit time-related changes associated with exposure to the drug.
- Multiple Studies Combined: The developers may conduct a smaller study labeled as a pilot study to determine the population size required to achieve at least 80% power. In most instances, choosing a population with a narrow demographic will reduce the population size requirement, such as age, gender, BMI, race, and other factors available. The PK/PD data are not likely to be available in the public domain data for the reference product since that would have been tested in a more diverse population. If a follow-up study is required and the developer can match the study population, use the duplicate lots of proposed biological products and reference products. The additional study(ies) data can be combined to conduct the final bioequivalence analysis. The developers are advised to secure the agency's approval before conducting a follow-up study.
- Unified Study: The developers may consider a study design that combines the PK and PD studies with clinical immunogenicity testing to minimize exposure to test subjects. For example, a two-arm parallel study with two dose levels and a follow-up after the second (higher) dose to study immunogenic attributes may suffice. However, to establish sufficient power, the developers must justify the study size, criteria for selecting subjects, and doses.
- Study Materials: All clinical pharmacology studies should be performed using proposed biological product materials from the final manufacturing process expected to be used for the marketed product if marketing authorization is granted. All proposed biological products must be manufactured in only one site. A study may include more than one comparator, but each must be used in the entire study. The developers should know that the ICH Q5E considerations do not apply to biologicals while developing a proposed biological product.

3.7.3 PHARMACOKINETIC PARAMETERS

Bioequivalence studies are generally not required for generic chemical drug products administered by the subcutaneous or intravenous route since, by definition, they are considered 100% bioavailable. A bioequivalence test for generic drugs aims to compare the dosage form's properties to release the drug at the action site. Once a drug has been released, the rest of the drug's time course from a generic product will be the same as expected for the molecules from the reference product because a proposed biological product and the reference product are chemically identical. The study design of bioequivalence testing of a generic product is based on universal acceptance of variation (0.8, 1.25) because this testing is *not* intended to compare the product's safety or efficacy—both of which are already established.

The testing of the PK profile of the proposed biological product against the reference product uses the same premise as the testing for generic chemical drugs because, just like the chemical generics, the purpose is to establish efficacy based on overall exposure that depends on the disposition profile that may vary because of subtle differences in the chemical structure of the molecule, differences in clearance induced by differences in immunogenic response and other factors that might alter safety and efficacy of a proposed biological product.

In those instances where the products are administered by routes other than intravenous, there may be differences in the absorption rates such as the subcutaneous route. Still, in most cases, these will not be significant. However, where a delayed or prolonged absorption is anticipated, the PK profile will be appropriate for determining the differences, examples include long-acting insulin products.

The equivalence criteria (0.8, 1.25) can be challenged by the developers with justification. The PK is used to detect possible differences in the interaction with the body between the reference product and a proposed biological product within a pre-specified acceptance range that may need modification. The location and the confidence interval's width should also be considered in the interpretation of similarity. For example, statistically significant differences in 90% of CIs within the justified acceptance range regarding relevant PK parameters would need to be explained and justified not to preclude biosimilarity. On the other hand, if the 90% CI crosses the prespecified boundaries, the developers would need to explain such differences and explore root causes. Correction for protein content may be acceptable on a case-by-case basis if pre-specified and adequately justified. The results from the assay of the test and reference product are included in the protocol.

All PK measures should be obtained for both a proposed biological product and the reference product. In a single-dose PK study, the primary parameters are the $AUC_{(0-inf)}$ for intravenous administration and $AUC_{(0-inf)}$ and usually C_{max} for subcutaneous administration. Secondary parameters, such as t_{max}, the volume of distribution, and half-life, should also be estimated. In a multiple-dose study, the primary parameters should be the truncated AUC after the first administration until the second administration (AUC_{0-t}) and AUC over a steady-state dosage interval (AUC_{0-ss}). Secondary parameters are C_{max} and C_{trough} at a steady state. The $AUC_{0-\infty} = AUC_{0-t} + C_t/Kel$ (or C_t (concentration at the last measurable time point) divided by Kel (elimination rate constant)) is calculated based on an appropriate method. C_{max} should be determined from the data without interpolation.

TABLE 3.4
Relevant Pharmacokinetic Parameters

Parameter	Significance
C_{max}	Rate of absorption, reaching minimum adequate levels (dose and drug delivery system
T_{max}	Rate of absorption with minimal impact on disposition because of faster absorption from parenteral administration (dose and delivery system)
$AUC_{0-inf,0-ss,0-t}$	Absorption, distribution, and elimination (structural difference, dose dependence)
V_{dss}	Distribution, receptor binding (structural differences)
dV_{dss}/dt	The thermodynamic potential of molecules to interact with tissue receptors, distribute, and bind due to structural differences
$AUCV_d$	Distribution, receptor binding (structural differences, dose)
K_{el}	Metabolism (structural differences, dose dependence)

For intravenous studies, $AUC_{0-\infty}$ will be considered the primary endpoint. For subcutaneous studies, C_{max} and AUC will be considered co-primary study endpoints. For multiple-dose studies, the total exposure measurement should be the area under the concentration–time profile from time zero to the end of the dosing interval at steady-state (AUC_{0-tau}) and is considered the primary endpoint. The concentration before the next dose during multiple dosing ($C_{trough\ ss}$) and C_{max} are considered secondary endpoints. Population PK data will not provide an adequate assessment of PK similarity.

In any PK study, anti-drug antibodies (ADAs) should be measured parallel to PK assessment using appropriate sampling time points.

Table 3.4 lists the PK parameters and their significance.

3.7.4 New Approach to PK Analysis

The PK parameters described above are commonly used to compare PK profiles. However, an emerging approach involves a thermodynamic assessment of the time course of a drug in the body based on the distribution volume. The apparent volume of distribution (V_d) is an important pharmacokinetic parameter that relates drug plasma concentrations to the amount of drug in the body and is essential for drug loading dose and maintenance dose calculations. Following an intravenous bolus of a drug, the volume of distribution of a drug varies with time. This redistribution occurs in two distinct phases with very different time scales: an avascular phase and a washout or dilution phase. During the vascular phase, a drug mixes throughout the blood's plasma volume with a time scale of seconds or minutes. During the dilution phase, hydrophilic drugs are distributed into the body's interstitial fluids with a time scale of hours or days. While most drugs are actively redistributing from plasma into the body tissues, the decrease in plasma concentrations is mainly due to that redistribution instead of actual drug elimination. In the following, we assume first-order kinetics, i.e., that drug elimination is proportional to its concentration, which is the most common drug kinetic. The most calculated volumes of distribution are the apparent volume of drug distribution immediately after intravenous bolus injection, i.e., at time zero (V_0), the evident terminal volume of distribution following bolus intravenous administration (V_{area}), and the expected volume of distribution, V_{ss} that is the apparent terminal volume of distribution, analogous to V_{area} in a bolus model. V_{ss} is the expected physical volume of distribution of the drug for bolus experiments, and unlike V_{ss}, it is invariant between constant infusion and bolus experiments.

A thermodynamic approach to using the volume of distribution involves a temporally variable, apparent volume of distribution model for the sum of exponential functions based on the conservation of mass. This variable volume model implies an explicit relationship between redistribution and the rate of volume of drug distribution expansion in time. Such a model specifies when the drug volume reaches a particular size relative to its apparent terminal distribution volume. Such a variable volume model could potentially provide unanticipated new information about time-based tissue drug effects for tissue metabolism and elimination. This model also has implications for the effects of drugs on body tissues, i.e., therapeutic, toxic, or radiation exposure effects.

A variable volume model could be used to calculate the optimal instantaneous dose that will produce a desired concentration at the effector site without an overload of the drug. A time-dependent apparent volume of distribution model based on mass conservation could be used with almost any concentration washout fit function. The distribution parameters can be sensitive to biological drugs that act by receptor binding, and the elimination constant can be more sensitive to structural variants leading to differences in the degradation of the administered drug; the appropriate parameters to include in a PK study are Vd_{ss} as a function of time besides other Vd parameters.

The elimination rate constant, $K_{el,}$ obtained from the terminal portion of the curve, or the half-life, is sensitive to how the body disposes of the molecules; structural differences not possible to quantify using traditional methods may show differences in the metabolism of the administered drug, and this parameter should be considered a pivotal consideration.

3.7.5 PK/PD Waivers

Although the comparison of target-mediated clearance is essential in the biosimilarity exercise, it may not be feasible in patients due to significant variability in target expression, including variability over time. However, since *in vitro* studies are expected to show comparable interaction between a proposed biological product and its target(s) (including FcRn for a mab), the absence of a pivotal PK study in the target population is acceptable if additional PK data are collected during the efficacy, safety, and PD studies as this allows further investigation of the clinical impact of variable pharmacokinetics and possible changes in the PK over time. This can be achieved by determining the PK profile in a subset of patients or population pharmacokinetics.

Comparative pharmacokinetic studies are a basic requirement for proposed biological development and are usually more sensitive than clinical efficacy trials when detecting potential product-related differences. This may explain why a demonstration of equivalent efficacy does not overrule a finding of dissimilar pharmacokinetic profiles.

Comparative efficacy studies are no longer deemed necessary for several product categories (insulin, low-molecular-mass heparins, and (peg)filgrastim), for which pivotal evidence for similarity may be derived from physicochemical, functional, PK, and PD comparisons. Exceptions to this include complex, multifunctional biologicals, where comparative efficacy and safety clinical trials in patients, are still viewed as a necessary component of proposed biological development.

3.7.5.1 Route of Administration

If the reference product can be administered intravenously and subcutaneously, the evaluation of subcutaneous administration will usually be sufficient to cover both absorption and elimination.

It is possible to waive the evaluation of intravenous administration if a proposed biological product appears comparative in both absorption and elimination for the subcutaneous route. The omission of the PK study of intravenous administration needs to be justified, e.g., when the molecule has an absorption constant much slower than the elimination constant (flip-flop kinetics).

While most biological drugs are administered systemically, a special case situation arises for drugs like ranibizumab, bevacizumab, and aflibercept administered intravitreally. Since the site of action is aqueous humor, this is the most desirable sampling site; the systemic testing shows that ranibizumab appears in the smallest concentration. It is cleared fast, followed in the rate by aflibercept and then bevacizumab. The developers are encouraged to develop an appropriate animal testing model using an *in-silico* approach to suggest waiving systemic PK/PD studies. Additionally, the direct immune response cannot be tested since ocular immune privilege protects the eye, significantly lowering immunogenic response. However, as the drug is cleared through systemic fluids, it is important to establish the ADA response.

3.7.6 PD PARAMETERS

A well-designed clinical PK and PD study in a proposed biological development program aims to evaluate the similarities and differences in the PK and PD profiles between a proposed biological product and the reference product. A well-designed clinical PK and PD study should include information about the exposure and, when possible, the exposure response to the biological products, which are essential for assessing whether there are any potential clinically meaningful differences between the two products. Determining the exposure response to a biological product can be particularly challenging because of biological products' complex nature and heterogeneity. Thus, the valuation of clinical pharmacology similarity should include assessments of PK similarity and, if applicable, PD similarity.

To the extent possible, the developers should select PD measures that (i) are relevant to clinical outcomes (e.g., on a mechanical path of MOA or disease process related to effectiveness or safety); (ii) are measurable for a sufficient period after dosing to ascertain the full PD response and with appropriate precision; and (iii) have the sensitivity to detect clinically meaningful differences between a proposed biological product and the reference product use of multiple PD measures that assess different domains of activities may also be of value.

The PD biomarker(s) used to measure PD response should be a single biomarker or a composite of biomarkers that effectively demonstrate the product's target effects' characteristics. Using a single scientifically appropriate PD biomarker or a composite of more than one relevant PD biomarker can reduce residual uncertainty regarding the existence of any clinically meaningful differences between products. It can significantly add to the overall demonstration of biosimilarity. Using broader panels of PD biomarkers (e.g., by conducting a protein or mRNA microarray analysis) that capture the product's multiple pharmacological effects can be of additional value. When determining which biomarkers should be used to measure response, it is important to consider the following five characteristics:

- The time of onset of change in the PD biomarker relative to dosing and its return to baseline with discontinuation of dosing.
- The dynamic range of the PD biomarker over the exposure range to the biological product.
- The sensitivity of the PD biomarker to differences between a proposed biological product and the Reference Product.
- The relevance of the PD biomarker to the mechanism of action of the drug (to the extent that the mechanism of action is known for the RP).
- The analytical validity of the PD biomarker assay

Sometimes, PD biomarkers with the relevant characteristics listed above are not identified. However, the developers are still encouraged to incorporate PD biomarkers that achieve a large dynamic range over the PK evaluation's concentration range because these PD biomarkers represent potential orthogonal tests that can support similarity.

When PD biomarkers are not sensitive or specific enough to detect clinically meaningful differences, the derived PK parameters should be used as the primary basis for evaluating similarity from a clinical pharmacology perspective. The PD biomarkers can be used to augment the PK data. A combination of PK and PD similarity can be an important assessment in demonstrating that there is no clinically meaningful difference between a proposed biological product and the reference product.

It is recommended that PD markers are added to the pharmacokinetic studies whenever feasible.

In some instances, comparative PK/PD studies may be sufficient to demonstrate a clinical comparative of a proposed biological product and the reference product, as enumerated below in the testing requirements.

- The selected PD marker/biomarker is an accepted surrogate marker. It can be related to the patient outcome to the extent that demonstrating a similar effect on the PD marker will ensure a similar effect on the clinical outcome. Relevant examples include an absolute neutrophil count to assess the effect of granulocyte-colony stimulating factor (G-CSF), early viral load reduction in chronic hepatitis C to assess the effect of alpha interferons, and euglycemic clamp test to compare two insulins. Magnetic resonance imaging of disease lesions can compare two β-interferons in multiple sclerosis.

- PD markers may not be established surrogates for efficacy but are relevant for the active substance's pharmacological action, and a clear dose–response or a concentration–response relationship has been demonstrated. In this case, a single- or multiple-dose-exposure-response study at two or more doses may be sufficient to waive a clinical efficacy study. This design would ensure that a proposed biological product and the reference can be compared within the dose–response curve's steep part.
- When there are established dose–response or systemic exposure–response relationships (response may be PD measures or clinical endpoints), it is important to select, whenever possible, a dose(s) for study on the steep part of the dose–response curve for a proposed biological product. Studying doses that are on the plateau of the dose–response curve is unlikely to detect differences between a proposed biological product and the reference product
- When evidence to establish comparative no clinically meaningful difference will be derived from PK studies supported by studies with non-surrogate PD/biomarkers, the plan should include a proposal of the size of the equivalence margin(s) with its clinical justification as well as of the measures for demonstration of a comparable safety profile.
- The selection of appropriate time points and durations for the measure of PD biomarkers will depend on the characteristics of the PD biomarkers (e.g., the PD response timing after the product's administration based on the product's half-life and the anticipated duration of the product's effect).
- When a PD response lags after initiation of product administration, a study of multiple-dose and steady-state conditions can be critical, primarily if a proposed therapy is intended for long-term use.
- The PD biomarker(s) evaluated for a proposed biological product and the reference product should be compared by determining the area under the effect curve. If only one PD measurement is available because of the characteristics of the PD biomarker, the measurement should be linked to a simultaneous drug concentration measurement. The relationship between drug concentration and the PD biomarker should then be used to compare products.
- Using a single, scientifically appropriate PD biomarker, as described above, or a composite of more than one relevant PD biomarker, can reduce any residual uncertainty about whether there are clinically meaningful differences between products and add significantly to the overall demonstration of biosimilarity. Using broader panels of biomarkers (e.g., by conducting a protein or mRNA microarray analysis) that capture multiple pharmacological effects of the product *can* also add value.
- For PD studies using products with a short half-life (e.g., shorter than 5 days), a rapid PD response, and a low incidence of immunogenicity, crossover design is appropriate when feasible. A parallel design is usually needed for products with a longer half-life (e.g., more than 5 days). The developers should provide a scientific justification for the selection of study dose (e.g., one dose or multiple doses) and route of administration.

- The optimal sampling strategy for determining PD measures can differ from the strategy used for PK measures. For PK sampling, frequent sampling at early time points following product administration with decreased frequency is generally most effective in characterizing the concentration–time profile. However, the PD–time profile might not mirror the PK–time profile. In such cases, the PD sampling should be well justified. When PK and PD data are obtained during a clinical pharmacology study, the sampling strategy should be optimized for both PK and PD measures.

3.8 CLINICAL IMMUNOGENICITY ASSESSMENT

Immunogenicity testing can be and preferably combined with PK/PD profiling; however, in some situations, an independent study must be conducted where a specific population or protocol is required that may not allow combining the study with PK/PD studies. The developers must first establish that there is no residual uncertainty regarding the factors responsible for immunogenicity response before conducting clinical testing. A more important element of these studies is the evaluation of ADAs that should be estimated from public domain data; for example, filgrastim has an extremely low immunogenic response, and pegylation of the molecules makes it even less immunogenic; therefore, any studies for filgrastim must provide for acceptance criteria that will have clinical meaningfulness. Recently, it has been determined that for simpler, low molecular weight products where the immunogenic response is not likely to affect clinical efficacy, immunogenicity studies will not be needed, such as in the case of insulin products. The developers may present challenges to conducting immunogenicity testing based on similar or other novel arguments.

The FDA has recently issued guidance removing the requirement to test the clinical immunogenicity of insulin if it meets analytical similarity testing; the factors responsible for this waiver are a smaller molecule with less complexity. More waivers of this type can be expected in the future.

Immunogenicity or adverse immune response is defined as the propensity of the therapeutic biologics to generate immune responses to itself and related proteins or induce immunologically related nonclinical effects or adverse clinical events. There are two types of immunogenicity in the therapeutic biologics development process:

- Wanted immunogenicity is typically related to vaccines. The injection of an antigen (the vaccine) stimulates an immune response against the pathogen (virus, bacteria, cancer cell, etc.), aiming at protecting the organism.
- Unwanted immune responses to therapeutic biologics may also neutralize their biological activities and result in adverse events not only by inhibiting the efficacy of the therapeutic biologics but also by cross-reacting to an endogenous protein counterpart, leading to loss of its physiological function (e.g., neutralizing antibodies to therapeutic erythropoietin cause pure red cell aplasia by also neutralizing the endogenous protein). This overview's meaning of immunogenicity is the latter adverse immune response in therapeutic biologics discovery and development.

The antigenic processes are performed by professional APCs such as DCs, macrophages, and B cells. There are two steps: first, the antigen capture that delivers antigens to the cellular antigen processing machinery, and second, the antigen processing and presentation that generates antigenic peptides bound to MHC molecules for presentation to adaptive immune cells. APCs capture the extracellular antigens through phagocytosis, macropinocytosis, and receptor-mediated endocytosis. In the acidic environment of endosomes or lysosomes, antigens are degraded into many immunogenic peptides that contain T-cell epitopes. Following antigens' intake, MHC class II molecular is synthesized in the endoplasmic reticulum and then transported by the Golgi apparatus to combine with antigen peptides to form peptide–MHC II complexes that are presented to the surface of APCs. TCR can recognize the peptide–MHC II complexes to activate T cells to initiate an immunogenic response. The antigen presentation's quality depends on the peptide–MHC complexes' affinity, and there is a direct relationship between peptide–MHC complex stability and the immunogenic response. Also, the binding ability between APCs and CD4+ T cells is determined by DC-T cell assay.

Immune responses to therapeutic biologics can significantly affect both efficacy and patient safety. The first-generation therapeutic mAbs were of murine origin, leading to highly adverse immune responses in patients because of the antibodies; much of these immunogenic responses are subdued in humanized mAbs, yet there remains a definite concern.

The adverse immune responses produce ADAs, which result in many clinically relevant effects (Table 3.5), leading to anaphylaxis, cytokine release syndrome, and cross-reactive neutralization of endogenous proteins mediating critical functions.

When ADAs have been demonstrated, further characterization beyond the titer and the antibodies' neutralizing capacity may be helpful, e.g., immunoglobulin class in acute hypersensitivity. It may also be possible to do further typing of clinically meaningful ADAs or determine a "threshold" level of ADAs beyond which there is a significant impact on efficacy and safety.

TABLE 3.5
Clinically Relevant Effects of Immunogenicity

Effects on bioavailability

Effect on safety and efficacy

Effect on PK, including potential cross-reactivity to endogenous proteins

Inhibition of the function of endogenous protein

Injection site reactions

Systemic reactions are mild or life-threatening

Formation of A.D.A. (HAMA, HACA, HAHA)

Formation of neutralizing antibodies

Formation of immune complexes

Formation of anti-idiotypic antibodies

TABLE 3.6
Immunogenicity Associated Factors

Category	Example
Treatment-associated	Mechanism of action
	Route of administration
	Frequency of administration, Duration of therapy
Patient-associated	Disease type
	Disease status
	Immune system function
	Genetic factors
	Concomitant disease
	Concomitant medications
	Prior exposure
	Prior sensitization
Drug property-associated	Recombinant expression system
	Post-translational protein modifications
	Impurities
	Contaminants
	Aggregates

Fundamentally, with therapeutic biologics being developed today, the most important factor concerning immunogenicity is that it is a covariate of pharmacokinetics; when immunogenicity against a therapeutic biologic occurs, it increases clearance and decreases exposure to that therapeutic. Both patient-related and product-related factors may affect the immunogenicity of therapeutic biologics. These factors are critical elements in the immunogenicity risk assessment (Table 3.6) and require consideration in immunogenicity testing protocols.

3.8.1   PK Dependence

The ADAs can influence pharmacokinetics, especially the elimination phase. Non-neutralizing, "binding" antibodies may sometimes also modulate rather than just decrease the efficacy of a product, e.g., by prolonging the half-life. A change in pharmacokinetics may be an early indication of antibody formation. Thus, the developers are encouraged to incorporate concomitant sampling for both pharmacokinetics and immunogenicity into all repeat dose studies.

3.8.2   Safety and Efficacy Correlation

The immunogenicity associated with intermittent treatment should be considered based on a risk assessment, e.g., experience from other similar products, risks associated with potential immunogenicity, boosting effect, and persistence or appearance of antibodies after the exposure.

The presence of ADAs may or may not have clinical consequences. It is essential that clinical development is based on an analysis of potential risks and possibilities to detect and mitigate them. The planning of the analysis of immune-mediated adverse effects (AEs) should be based on risk analysis, including previous experience with the product (class), potentially immunogenic structures in the protein, and patient population. Patients with pre-existing ADAs may exhibit a different efficacy and safety profile and should be analyzed as a subgroup when feasible. The analysis plan should define symptom complexes associated with acute or delayed hypersensitivity, autoimmunity, and loss of efficacy. Potential immunological AEs should be addressed in the risk management plan.

3.8.3 Management of Immunogenicity Testing

A harmful immune reaction to a therapeutic protein cannot always be avoided despite the developers' efforts to select compounds with low immunogenic potential. In such cases, the developers should, if feasible, explore possibilities to reduce the adverse impact of immunogenicity observed during clinical development. In some cases, immunosuppressive or anti-inflammatory co-medication may significantly prevent or mitigate adverse immunological effects. In some cases, as with coagulation factors, it may be possible to re-establish the immunological tolerance by tolerization regimens, e.g., by administering larger doses of a therapeutic protein. Clinical studies should document such therapeutic regimens.

3.9 CLINICAL EFFICACY ASSESSMENT

The BPCIA states: "If there is residual uncertainty about biosimilarity after conducting structural analyses, functional assays, animal testing, human PK and PD studies, and the clinical immunogenicity assessment, the sponsor should then consider what additional clinical data may be needed to address that uncertainty adequately." The additional clinical study does not necessarily mean a clinical efficacy study; it could be extra in silico pharmacokinetic studies as suggested in the FDA's Biosimilar Action Plan. Therefore, we should establish the "residual uncertainty" after clinical pharmacology studies have been completed, avoiding "putting patients through all these different trials just to check a box."

According to the BPCIA, biosimilars "may be approved based on PK and PD biomarker data without a comparative clinical study with efficacy endpoint(s)." Reliance on PK and PD biomarker data in healthy subjects or patients allows for shorter and less costly clinical studies] and provides more sensitive testing than the clinical efficacy with endpoint(s). The PD biomarker(s) used to measure PD response can be a single biomarker or a composite of more than one relevant PD biomarker that effectively demonstrates the characteristics of the product's target effects. Using broader panels of PD biomarkers (e.g., by measuring features of the transcriptome, proteome, and epigenome), capturing multiple pharmacological effects of the product may be of additional value.

Clinical efficacy testing is conducted in equivalence or non-inferiority based on clinical response or endpoints. In the equivalence testing mode, first, we establish the M1 or total efficacy value of the reference product— a highly variable parameter, but available; second, we choose an acceptable range of difference, the M2, that is based on the clinical judgment that is difficult to be definitive—at best it is an arbitrary choice.

As a result, the equivalence studies are least likely to fail because both products are supposed to be equivalent. So far, no equivalence study for biosimilars has resulted in the rejection of biosimilarity. The fact is that a comparative study for two products that are anticipated to be identical is highly unlikely to be discriminatory because the dosing is inevitably at the plateau level, where a difference is unlikely to be recorded.

Comparative equivalence studies are required to have homogeneity of the study population, an unlikely possibility for many drugs, including anticancer drugs, where the patients are inevitably exposed to several drugs and treatment modalities; additionally, the anticancer drugs have a meager efficacy rate that further reduces the statistical probability of identifying any difference. Efficacy studies for oncology or other terminal illness drugs present unique challenges, including recruiting a comparable population, such as naïve patients. The short lifetime of patients disrupting the study design further makes such studies of little value.

Non-inferiority studies are discouraged because of the likelihood of approving a more effective biosimilar with higher toxicity since the two are proportional to biological drugs.

A misconception that lesser clinical evidence is needed if the product shows higher similarity in biological and physical–chemical assays is ill-founded—every testing is conducted under protocols that either fail or pass. Since clinical efficacy testing cannot support the validity of biological and chemical assays, any concessions made in clinical efficacy testing are not valid.

Generally, "additional clinical studies may be required" if residual uncertainty remains after completing the analytical assessment, nonclinical, and clinical pharmacology studies. Whereas in most cases, a single study in one of several approved indications may be sufficient to establish biosimilarity, but where multiple modes of action are involved, a single study in one indication alone may or may not be enough to remove "residual uncertainty." the developers are strongly urged to consult with agencies before conducting clinical efficacy testing to make sure that the selected protocol is suitable to remove identified residual uncertainty(ies).

3.9.1 RESIDUAL UNCERTAINTY

After completing all the above-listed testing, the developer should prepare a detailed justification to demonstrate to the agency that a proposed biological product has the required biosimilarity to allow licensing (in the US) or authorization (in other countries). This is the most critical stage where a developer can save 24–36 months and scores of millions of dollars from securing approval. Most proposed biological developers are too eager to jump to safety and efficacy studies to support their marketing efforts based on their archaic understanding of selling biological drugs through prescribers. Suppose the developer can demonstrate no residual uncertainty in a strong argument. In that case, any additional clinical testing will not be required, and even if it is, this may be limited to further clinical pharmacology studies.

The developers should argue that the totality of the evidence provided is sufficient to determine that a proposed biological product is proposed biological to the reference product. The arguments should include a description of any differences in the analytical, nonclinical, and clinical pharmacology assessments in this specific order, realizing that a residual uncertainty must be removed (either proving it nonconsequential or demonstrating that it does not impact clinical safety and efficacy). One argument favoring the developer is that additional testing may not remove any marginal residual uncertainty.

As a scientific matter, a comparative clinical study will be necessary to support a demonstration of biosimilarity if there is residual uncertainty about whether there are clinically meaningful differences between a proposed biological product and the reference product based on structural and functional characterization, animal testing, human PK and PD data, and clinical immunogenicity assessment. The developers should provide a scientific justification if they believe a comparative clinical study is unnecessary.

A proposed biological product tested stepwise undergoes identification and removal of residual uncertainty at each step before moving forward to another testing in the following order: analytical, functional, in vitro, in vivo, clinical pharmacology, and immunogenicity. While most biological developers routinely conduct clinical efficacy testing as listed in Appendix 3, Agencies consider unnecessary patient exposure inappropriate and encourage them to meet with Agencies to understand what they consider as the remaining residual uncertainty.

In most cases, at this stage of development, a failed PK/PD/Immunogenicity testing will reject a proposed biological product for a proposed biological status. The developer may choose to refile the applications as a new biological drug. The residual uncertainties identified at this stage are structural, functional, or nonclinical testing, where the variation may not be evaluated thoroughly for impact on safety and efficacy.

3.9.2 WAIVERS

With suitable PD endpoints and a clear understanding of the mechanism of action, a PK/PD study may be sufficient clinical work for marketing authorization. However, comparative efficacy and safety clinical trials in patients are still considered necessary components of proposed biological development for complex, multifunctional biologicals. The need for testing in patients is driven by the often-unresolvable complexity of interactions resulting from the size of the molecule, diverse moieties with different functions (e.g., Fab/Fc-parts), multiple mechanisms of action, the impact of glycosylation pattern, and potential for immunogenicity and potentially life-threatening AEs).

As more proposed biological product is approved globally and safety and efficacy data are becoming available to regulatory agencies, a trend is developing to question comparative efficacy testing relevance. Agencies expect the developers to adduce arguments in favor of avoiding clinical efficacy testing that does not result in a meaningful comparison, expose patients to avoidable risks, and does not establish a bridge between any multiple indications approved for the reference product

In most cases, a comparative clinical study is essential to rule out clinically meaningful differences in efficacy and safety between a proposed biological product and the reference product. A clinical efficacy trial may not always be necessary, e.g., a clinically relevant PD endpoint. In such cases, a scientific justification is needed to conduct an efficacy study, yet the safety and comparative immunogenicity data are still required.

3.9.3 SELECTION OF STUDY PROTOCOLS

The comparative clinical study should be adequately sensitive to rule out clinically meaningful differences within predefined comparability margins. The developers should consider the following factors when designing an adequately sensitive clinical study:

- The characteristics of the studied population(s) (e.g., underlying disease and immune competence).
- The clinical studies' characteristics include study duration, route of administration, dosage regimen, clinical endpoint(s), and assessment time.
- The risk and impact of immunogenicity.
- The impact of concomitant therapies (e.g., monotherapy vs. combination therapy).
- The use of appropriate comparability margins.

In some instances, evaluating more than one sensitive population may be necessary.
    The following are examples of factors that may influence the type and extent of the comparative clinical study data needed:

- The nature and complexity of the reference product, the extensiveness of structural and functional characterization, and the findings and limitations of comparative structural, functional, and nonclinical testing, including the extent of observed differences.
- The extent to which differences in structure, function, and nonclinical pharmacology and toxicology predict differences in clinical outcomes, in conjunction with the degree of understanding of the MOA of the reference product and disease pathology.
- The extent to which human PK or PD is known to predict clinical outcomes (e.g., PD measures known to be relevant to effectiveness or safety).
- The extent of clinical experience with the reference product and its therapeutic class, including the safety and risk–benefit profile (e.g., whether there is a low potential for off-target adverse events) and appropriate endpoints and biomarkers for safety and effectiveness (e.g., availability of established, sensitive clinical endpoints).
- The extent of any other clinical experience with a proposed biological product.

The developers should provide a scientific justification for how they intend to use these factors to determine what type(s) of clinical study are needed and any necessary study design. For example, suppose a comparative clinical study is needed.

In that case, the developers should explain how these factors were considered in determining a study's design, including the endpoint(s), population, similarity margin, and statistical analyses.

Additionally, specific safety or effectiveness concerns regarding the reference product and its class (including the history of manufacturing- or source-related adverse events) may warrant more comparative clinical data. Alternatively, suppose there is information regarding other biological products that could support a biosimilarity determination (with marketing histories demonstrating no apparent differences in clinical safety and effectiveness profiles). In that case, such information may help a selective and targeted approach to the clinical program.

Without surrogate markers for efficacy, it is usually necessary to demonstrate comparable clinical efficacy of a proposed biological product and the reference product in an adequately powered, randomized, parallel-group comparative clinical study(s), preferably double-blind, using efficacy endpoints. The study population should represent the reference product's approved therapeutic indication(s) and be sensitive to detecting potential differences between a proposed biological product and the reference. Occasionally, clinical practice changes may require a deviation from the approved therapeutic indication, e.g., a concomitant medication used in combination treatment, line of therapy, or disease severity. Deviations need to be justified and discussed with regulatory authorities.

3.9.3.1   Study Design

Careful consideration should be given to the study's design, including the choice of primary efficacy endpoints and comparative clinical margins. Each of these aspects is important and should be justified on clinical grounds. The study should use a clinically relevant and sensitive endpoint to show no clinically meaningful difference between a proposed biological product and the reference product. The chosen endpoint could differ from the original study endpoint for the reference product (e.g., a well-established surrogate or a more sensitive endpoint). An acceptable comparability margin should be defined in all cases, considering the smallest effect size that the reference product would reliably be expected to have based on publicly available historical data. If multiple endpoints are used, then the principles described above should apply.

In line with the principle of similarity, equivalence trials are generally preferred. If non-inferiority trials are considered, they should be justified, and the developer is advised to consult with Agencies before study initiation. The developers should be aware that such trials' results could suggest a proposed biological product's statistical superiority relative to the reference product. In such instances, the superiority observed should be assessed for clinical relevance, including its impact on safety. If the superiority observed is clinically meaningful and is associated with increased adverse drug reactions over those seen with the reference product, the product would no longer be considered biological. Also, the demonstration of non-inferiority of a proposed biological product to the reference product might not provide strong support for the authorization of other indications, particularly if the other indications include different dosages than those tested in the clinical study.

3.9.3.2   Efficacy Endpoints

In a comparative clinical study, the developers should use endpoints to assess clinically meaningful differences between a proposed biological product and the reference product. The endpoints may differ from those used as primary endpoints in the RP's clinical studies if they are scientifically supported. Specific endpoints (such as PD measures) are more sensitive than clinical endpoints and may enable more precise comparisons of relevant therapeutic effects. When assessing multiple PD measures in a comparative clinical study, there may be situations that will enhance the study's sensitivity. The adequacy of the endpoints depends on the extent to which PD measures correlate with clinical outcome, the extent of structural and functional data support for biosimilarity, the understanding of MOA, and the nature or seriousness of the outcome affected.

While the hard clinical outcome remains the most desirable endpoint, other clinical endpoints that require shorter study times have been widely used (Table 3.7).

The developers should justify that the chosen model is relevant and sensitive to detect potential efficacy and safety differences. Differences detected between the efficacy of a proposed biological product and a reference product should always be discussed as to whether they are clinically relevant. Generally, clinical data aim to address slight differences observed in previous steps and confirm the comparable clinical performance of a proposed biological product and the reference product. Clinical data cannot be used to justify substantial differences in quality attributes.

Comparative margins should be prespecified and justified on both statistical and clinical grounds by using the reference product's data and all comparative clinical study designs and assay sensitivity. See ICH topic E9 Statistical principles for clinical studies and CHMP guideline CPMP/EWP/2158/99 on the choice of the noninferiority margin.

TABLE 3.7
Clinical Endpoints in Proposed Biological Testing

Absolute neutrophil count for granulocyte-colony stimulating factor (G-CSF)

Blood glucose concentrations in clamp studies for insulins

Complete pathological response (pCR) in breast cancer

Disease Activity Score [D.A.S.]-28 versus American College of Rheumatology-20 in rheumatoid arthritis Disease

Objective response rate in solid tumors and lymphoma

Factor X and anti-Factor II activity, Magnetic resonance imaging-related endpoints for interferon-β,

Use of serum calcium levels for teriparatide

Bone mineral density together with serum C-terminal crosslinks, a bone resorption marker, as co-primary efficacy endpoints for denosumab to treat and prevent osteoporosis

α4-integrin receptor saturation for natalizumab as the binding is directly linked to clinical outcomes Serum lactate dehydrogenase levels and for eculizumab.

3.10   EXTRAPOLATION OF CLINICAL DATA ACROSS INDICATIONS

Suppose a proposed biological product meets the biosimilarity and other regulatory requirements for marketing authorization as a proposed biological product based on, among other things, data derived from a clinical study or studies sufficient to demonstrate safety, purity, and potency in an appropriate condition of use. In that case, the developers must seek marketing authorization for a proposed biological product for one or more additional conditions of use for which the reference product is authorized.

However, the developers would need to provide sufficient scientific justification for extrapolating clinical data to determine biosimilarity for each condition of use for which marketing authorization is sought.

Such scientific justification for extrapolation should address, for example, the following issues for the tested and extrapolated conditions of use:

- The MOA (s) in each condition of use for which marketing authorization is sought may include the following:
  The target/receptor(s) for each relevant activity/function of the product.
  The binding, dose/concentration-response, and pattern of molecular signaling upon engagement of target/receptor(s).
  The relationships between product structure and target/receptor interactions.
  The location and expression of the target/receptor(s).
- The PK and bio-distribution of the product in different patient populations (Relevant PD measures may also provide important information on the MOA.).
- The immunogenicity of the product in different patient populations.
- Differences in expected toxicities in each condition of use and patient population (including whether expected toxicities are related to the pharmacological activity of the product or off-target activities).
- Any other factor that may affect the safety or efficacy of the product in each condition of use and patient population for which marketing authorization is sought.

Differences between conditions of use concerning the factors described above do not necessarily preclude extrapolation. A scientific justification should address these differences in the totality-of-the-evidence context, supporting a demonstration of biosimilarity.

In choosing which condition of use to study that would permit subsequent extrapolation of clinical data to other conditions of use, it is recommended that the developers consider choosing a condition of use that would be adequately sensitive to detect clinically meaningful differences between a proposed biological product and the reference product

The developers of a proposed biological product must obtain marketing authorization for all conditions of use previously approved for the reference product at the time of application. If the reference product receives marketing authorization for additional indications, the developers must add those indications before or after marketing authorization. However, if an indication is protected under IP laws, the developers may request fewer and add more indications as the IP expiration allows them.

The reference product may have more than one therapeutic indication. When biosimilarity in a comparative study has been demonstrated in one indication, extrapolation of clinical data to other indications of the reference product could be acceptable but needs to be scientifically justified. If it is unclear whether the safety and efficacy confirmed in one indication would be relevant for another indication, additional data will be required. Extrapolation should be considered in the light of the totality of data, i.e., quality, nonclinical, and clinical data. The safety and efficacy are expected to be extrapolated when thorough physicochemical and structural analyses have demonstrated proposed biological comparative and *in vitro* functional tests complemented with clinical data (efficacy and safety and PK/PD data) in one therapeutic indication. Additional data are required in certain situations, such as

- The active substance of the reference product interacts with several receptors that may have a different impact on the tested and non-tested therapeutic indications.
- The active substance itself has more than one active site, and the sites may have a different impact on different therapeutic indications.
- The studied therapeutic indication is not relevant for the others in terms of efficacy or safety, i.e., it is not sensitive to differences in all relevant aspects of efficacy and safety.

Immunogenicity is related to multiple factors, including the route of administration, dosing regimen, patient-related factors, and disease-related factors (e.g., co-medication, type of disease, and immune status). Thus, immunogenicity could differ among indications. Extrapolation of immunogenicity from the studied indication/route of administration to other uses of the reference product should be justified.

3.10.1 Additional Conditions of Use

Agencies recognize that a proposed biological product application holder may be interested in seeking marketing authorization for an additional condition(s) of use after product-market authorization. While this option is generally available in many jurisdictions, agencies allow a proposed biological product to add any new indications to the reference product in the future, provided no changes were made to the reference product. If an indication is protected under a patent, it is up to the developers to judge whether it is applicable in its region and solely responsible for litigation. Marketing authorization by agencies does not constitute an opinion regarding intellectual property associated with the reference product.

3.11 INTERCHANGEABILITY AND SUBSTITUTION

A generic drug is generally considered interchangeable with its reference (brand name) drug and other generic products that use the same reference drug. However, because a proposed biological is not structurally identical to its brand-name biologic, assessing interchangeability is a separate process. The FDA regulates drug products in the United States, but the states regulate pharmacies and pharmacy practices. According to the National Conference of State Legislatures (NCSL), as of October 22, 2018, "all states have established for substituting a proposed biological prescription product to replace an original biologic product."

The FDA has issued its final guidance on demonstrating the interchangeability of a proposed biological with its reference product to assist sponsors in showing that a proposed therapeutic protein product is interchangeable with the reference product. It is important to reiterate that the FDA guidelines are not binding, and for the same reason, they do not preclude a sponsor from making an alternate proposal to the FDA, even though most sponsors would hesitate to do so. FDA has approved several interchangeable products.

3.11.1 POST MARKET SURVEILLANCE

While a pharmacovigilance program will not satisfy any residual uncertainty in biosimilarity, in some cases, pharmacovigilance may provide additional confidence to regulatory agencies; for example, if the formation of ADAs is dependent on the demographic aspects, only a large study can provide a reliable data, and such information can be collected in a pharmacovigilance plan, among other routine and common attributes.

4 Optimization of Cost of Goods

4.1 BACKGROUND

A complete grasp of the manufacturing platform for therapeutic proteins requires a comprehension of the roles that DNA and RNA play in human bodies. The manufacturing processes are intimately connected to each unit activity of both upstream and downstream processing. The three main factors influencing each step are yield variability, variety of contaminants, and potency reached.

At the start of the manufacturing train, a modified genetically modified cell culture is generated to express the intended therapeutic protein in a bioreactor. [Terms fermenter and bioreactor are often used interchangeably; a fermenter is a bioreactor that generates heat and gases, while a bioreactor is a device to develop any form of live creature. Therapeutic proteins are better referred to as bioreactors.] Subsequently, the produced therapeutic protein must be extracted from the culture media. This can be achieved using filtration (if the protein is in solution) or a multi-step method that involves firstly disturbing the cells, such as bacteria, and then extracting the protein. As soon as the intended therapeutic protein is expressed (i.e., produced) by the living beings, this procedure starts. The next steps are the purification of the therapeutic proteins and, in some cases, the proper folding. It is imperative to eradicate any viral contaminations, particularly when the expression entities are mammalian cells that harbor viruses. The therapeutic protein is now prepared for labeling as a drug substance after it has been diluted in a buffer and maintained at -20 C. It is next processed to create a drug product, which can be a solution in a vial or prefilled syringe, or it can be a lyophilized powder. Currently, therapeutic proteins are administered parenterally, intravenously, or subcutaneously, but additional delivery methods such as oral, transdermal, inhalation, or others may become available in the future.

4.2 CREATION OF CELL LINES

The development of conventional cell lines starts with a tedious procedure. From conception to creation, a high-yielding, high-quality clone in early-stage manufacturing can take more than 40 weeks. This comprises choosing the right cell line, constructing an expression vector, transfection, cell sorting, and choosing and grading clones based on their growth and productivity. Single-cell isolation and screening are crucial phases in the cell-line development process from a regulatory perspective. The conventional screening procedure involves seeding a 96-well plate with one cell per well, screening multiple of these plates, and choosing a high producer.

Many methods are now available that can help reduce overall timeframes by expediting specific steps in the cell-line creation process. In contrast to the random

DOI: 10.1201/9781003404637-4

transfection events of the past, cell-line makers may now effectively employ a targeted transfection method that places the gene into "hot zones." This specific modification allows for the development of a high-producing cell line while significantly reducing the requirement for extra screening procedures. Additionally, by first sorting cells into mini-pools and then selecting a high-performing pool of cells, a smaller population can select the final single clone instead of screening multiple plates. This contrasts with screening each clone individually (50–100 in traditional processes). Combining fluorescence-activated cell sorting (FACS) with glutamine synthetase can further speed up the clone screening processes (FACS). These days, cell-line makers make substantial use of microfluidics-based technology. These technologies not only sort and deposit single cells to demonstrate proof of clonality, but they can also offer specific productivities and proliferation rates rapidly (as little as 5 days). Combining these technologies can reduce the time required to grow a cell line from 8 to 10 weeks, which can expedite process development and lead to early-stage deliverables.

Conventional approaches like plating into semi-solid media and detecting a clone's protein titer during the static phase are still highly valued by many producers, despite their poor association with fed-batch. For pre-selection, novel methods include vector optimization and FACS; enrichment for potentially higher producers is also a possibility.

In bioprocess technology, it's a prevalent misperception that you need to coerce the cell line to produce higher yields. This can only be carried only so far until the cell line becomes unstable; if the antibody is monoclonal, then variations in glycosylation and other DNA-based modifications will unavoidably take place despite the high titer it can produce. Developers must first calculate the cost of producing their product using the media that provides the carbon source, before switching to cell lines with greater yields. While a higher-yielding cell line typically helps reduce the bioreactor's size, it does not always result in a cheaper final product.

4.2.1 MEDIA

Cell culture media, which comes in over 100 formulations with different critical elements such as lipids, vitamins, fatty acids, and amino acids, is the primary basic material. How efficiently the media promotes protein quality, productivity, cellular metabolism, and cell development depends in large part on its composition, concentration, and chemical definition. Improvements in cell culture media have a significant effect on increased specific productivity, cell density, and product quality (less variability). This section discusses certain challenges and media optimization strategies that can enhance process intensification.

Media optimization approaches cannot be applied consistently to multiple cell lines or even clones; for instance, a media that boosts productivity in one clone could not have the same effect on another. This could also have an impact on the product's quality. Platform methods, particularly those that rely solely on one basal media, are never going to yield satisfactory outcomes. Even though using an existing media for all mAb products using the same host cell line may have advantages (e.g., ease of sourcing media components, a fixed and validated approach to preparation), variations in the product quality (e.g., glycosylation, charge variants) may be required for the functionality of the final product. For this reason, having unique solutions, even with a limited number of compounds, is highly recommended.

Typically, while creating a new medium and assessing if it is appropriate for a particular cell line, one media component is altered at a time. A Design of Experiment (DoE) technique enables the investigation of the interactions and effects of components to optimize the composition. It may take a long since, depending on the number of components being used, there may be multiple iterations. Due to its ability to optimize many components' media simultaneously, media blending is being used more and more as a replacement for traditional DoE procedures. Moreover, efficient media production requires precise analytical methods for measuring metabolites during the entire culture. For this, capillary electrophoresis (CE), HPLC in conjunction with MS, and GC are commonly used.

Contemporary technologies, including high throughput microarray analysis, evaluate these ions and metabolites independently; rather, they take a comprehensive approach to media analysis. When medium components that cells respond to are identified by microarray analysis, random testing is avoided (provided by EMD Millipore Sigma). Many cell culture media providers work with pharmaceutical companies to optimize media by offering high throughput technologies (e.g., Millipore Sigma, Sartorius). The media production industry can save a great deal of time and money by using modeling instead of additional research or even experimental analysis. In order to improve media or even feed solutions and create a more reliable process, these models can benefit from online or inline analysis conducted during cell culture. This is particularly valid for models that are stoichiometric and kinetic. Because of this, companies may choose to create platform cell culture media specifically for their own cell lines.

Most optimized cell culture media are made for fed-batch techniques that require sporadic feeding (mostly concentrates of specific media components). However, because perfusion culture requires enormous volumes of media, having an affordable media solution becomes even more important. Concentrating on cell culture medium is one tactic to reduce operational footprint. Volumes of around 60,000–70,000 L can be obtained by the concentrated medium at three to four times its component levels, easily supporting a perfusion process and saving a significant amount of space and resources. Another method to meet the criteria of the perfusion process media is to have media made especially for the procedure. This will be more appropriate to support high-cell densities, boost volumetric productivity, and reduce costs than changing the media used for a fed-batch process (lower perfusion rates) (Table 4.1).

Make advantage of Table 4.1 decision matrix to identify bottlenecks and create a next-generation procedure.

4.2.2   INCREASED DENSITY PRESERVATION OF CELLS

The process of creating a cell bank is the ideal candidate for process intensification. Before starting the cell banking process, a vial is usually thawed to inoculate at least a 25 mL culture. Subsequently, the culture is expanded to yield an enough quantity of cells for storage. Vials with about a million cells have been used by the industry in general. In comparison to a production bioreactor operating on a commercial

TABLE 4.1
Next Generation Matrix to Address Bottlenecks and New Processes

Technology Solution	Pros	Cons	Comment
Bottleneck: Limited Facility Foot Print			
Perfusion	High volumetric productivity	Operational complexity	Needs more process development than fed-batch
Bottleneck: Limited CAPEX			
Perfusion	Smaller bioreactor	Operational complexity	Needs more process development than fed-batch
Bottleneck: Limited Capacity in Production Bioreactor			
N-1 perfusion	Cell expansion time shifts to N-1; shorter N time with same titer	Operational complexity, possible impact on process performance	Ensure capacity for shorter turn-around times
Perfusion	High volumetric productivity	Operational complexity	Identify a separation technique that will suit your process
Bottleneck: QC/QA Release			
Online sensors and PAT implementations	Reduce number of release methods through tighter process control	Resource demanding to develop	E.g. spectral methods combined with multivariant analysis can offer several process parameters
Multi-attribute re-lease methods	Drastic reduction of release methods	Resource demanding to develop	Still in development
Bottleneck: Low-Yield Process			
Perfusion	High volumetric productivity	Operational complexity	Identify a separation technique that will suit your process
Concentrated fed-batch	High volumetric productivity	Operational complexity	
Bottleneck: Several products and processes			
Perfusion	Higher level of flexibility	Operational complexity	Scale-out depending on batch volume needed

scale, the scale-up factor, or the number of seed trains required to create adequate inoculum from the vial to the production bioreactor, is larger. The process of creating seeds takes a long time, and additional tools and safety measures may be required. During the seed multiplication stage, moving from a low-density bank to a production bioreactor can take 20–30 days. To counteract this additional processing time, a high cell density bank that provides a larger working volume upon thaw is beginning to gain popularity. A high cell density cell bank can be added to the initial seed train bioreactor (N-3 bioreactor) as a means of reducing the inoculation time. For example, the seed expansion period can be shortened from 10 days to 2 weeks using a 100–150-mL high-density cell bag that has been cryopreserved and contains 50–100×106 cells/mL. This new technique minimizes variability in cell density, lowers the danger of contamination, and—most importantly—slashes the time required to start a production bioreactor. It also eliminates the need to handle many vials. For high cell density cryopreservation, a specific kind of medium is advised, one that can sustain high cell densities without resulting in any damage to the cells during freeze-thaw cycles. Additionally, state-of-the-art technologies are being developed to produce single-use bag assemblies in huge quantities for banking and cell freezing (fluoropolymer 2D bags).

4.2.3 Methods for Cell Culture

For the past few decades, fed-batch cultures have been the main emphasis. Large amounts of fluid and vessel capacity are needed for high cell densities and increased productivity, which is why perfusion systems are accessible but not widely used in the industry. Because of advancements made in increasing productivities, fed-batch has persisted for a very long period even though it can attain far lower cell densities than perfusion. The increasing adoption of single-use technologies is driving the development of perfusion-based processes, especially concentrated fed-batch, and steady-state perfusion in response to the requirement to lower costs of production and improve facility flexibility. Perfusion techniques can increase volumetric productivity in both the seed train and production periods by a factor of three. It is possible to accomplish upstream process intensification with perfusion-based methods. In order to enhance facility efficiency and usage, this means reducing the size and number of bioreactors required to minimize the seed train duration, maximizing bioreactor utilization, increasing volumetric output, and minimizing the overall footprint.

4.2.3.1 Perfusion

A kind of intensification known as N-1 perfusion refers to the quickening of cell growth in the phase before the production bioreactor (N). To attain maximum cell survival and density, this procedure The process of intensification involves attaching a cell retention device to the N-1 bioreactor. By doing this, the production bioreactor's run time is shortened and its starting cell density is increased. It can greatly increase the facility's output without substantially changing the main production process. A robust cell retention device is required to obtain a high cell density inoculum for the production bioreactor.

The following are some benefits of N-1 perfusion:

- Efficiency increases with the Fed-Batch approach
- Saved money and time
- reduced operational risk

- bioreactor footprint reduction
- N-1 perfusion can enhance Fed-batch output in two ways:
  - A high cell density is seeded into the production bioreactor (N) once the cell retention device is linked to the N-1 bioreactor.
  - The N-1 bioreactor with the cell retention device attached should be removed if the N-2 bioreactor can supply enough cells for the production bioreactor (N).

The most popular application in an N-1 bioreactor has been the use of perfusion. The N-1 bioreactor's cell density can be raised to start the production bioreactor with a high seeding density and possibly reduce the bioreactor's total cycle time to obtain the necessary titers. It is possible to inoculate many production bioreactors from a single N-1 bioreactor, which increases productivity and raises overall upstream capacity and production amounts. This increase in output can also be achieved with a reduced footprint; for example, the conventional approach requiring a 20,000 L bioreactor can now be replaced with a 2,000 L perfusion bioreactor. Furthermore, cleaning validation and CIP/SIP requirements are eliminated with the usage of single-use components. As was also previously indicated, the N-3 seed train and high cell density cryopreservation are additional steps down the perfusion-based method's hierarchy. By employing a single-use bag that can carry between 150 and 500 mL of high cell density culture, one can inoculate a seed bioreactor without the need for shake flasks or the laborious seed expansion procedure. After use, this bag can be frozen.

Perfusion can greatly increase cell density and speed up the production process in the N-1 bioreactor, leading to efficiency improvements. Adding perfusion culture to the seed train to increase cell density can reduce the number of bioreactors required or the time required to reach the target titer at harvest.

Process intensification can also be achieved through the use of concentrated fed-batch or intensified fed-batch modes. A concentrated fed-batch process recirculates the product and the cells, much like a perfusion technique does. The concentrated fed-batch method also makes use of the production bioreactor together with an ATF pump and hollow-fiber filter, just like perfusion does. However, in this case, the filter size should be adequate to retain both the product and the cells. When manufacturing antibodies, a 30-kDa filter is used. Usually, the procedure starts as a fed-batch operation and only starts to recycle the cells and product when the manufacturing cycle is almost over. Concentrated fed-batch procedures offer the benefit of high cell densities combined with the advantage of a single harvest operation—unlike perfusion—without titrating the product. The most well-known example of a concentrated fed-batch application is the Crucell and DSM project PERCIVIA. Based on the findings, the concentrated fed-batch approach yielded noticeably high yields of 27 g/L when PER.C6 cells were utilized.

This increased productivity, when paired with single-use technology (SUT), streamlines the procedure and permits the building of smaller facilities. A pharmaceutical manufacturer can boost their capacity to maintain competitiveness by incorporating these advantages into the existing framework.

4.3   BIOREACTOR CYCLE

One of a facility's primary production limitations is the production bioreactor. Since all other upstream and downstream process steps only take a few days at most, the length of the production bioreactor process—roughly 2 weeks for a fed-batch process—is frequently a rate-limiting step in an industrial facility. Thus, it is imperative to investigate the use of perfusion in the bioreactor immediately before production. The common end results include shorter processing durations, comparable titers, and higher densities during the inoculation stage of manufacturing. As a result, both the production process and the facility's total volumetric productivity have increased. Optimizing the perfusion medium to generate the necessary number of cells for the production bioreactor while avoiding adding to the already significant workload related to large-scale, irregular medium preparation in a facility is the second challenge. The primary determinants of the total mass of cells and products generated throughout the cell culture process are the cell densities obtained over time and the productivity of individual cells.

Upstream process intensification is also employed in the seed train. Here, an emerging strategy is to use perfusion instead of batches in the scale-up process. The objective is to develop a perfusion culture to an exceptionally high cell density, which can then be used to inoculate a production-scale reactor with very few intermediate scale-up stages. For example, a 10-L perfusion culture with 60 million cells/mL can be used to directly inoculate a 2,000-L reactor at an initial cell density of 0.3 million cells/mL. A more conventional scale-up strategy would have involved using batch cultures and intermediary vessels with capacities of, say, 50, 200, and 500 L. It is also feasible to inoculate the production culture at a high start cell concentration using a high-density seed culture. This can speed up the process and drastically cut down on the manufacturing lag time. A shorter process allows for higher annual production batches and better facility utilization. A description of perfusion is provided in order to improve the seed train. With the use of specially designed cryo bags, open cell culture operation steps can be eliminated, seed train expansion repeatability can be increased, batch production can be kept apart from cell expansion, and cells can be distributed globally to production facilities from a central expansion facility.

4.4   SINGLE-USE TECHNOLOGY (SUT)

Early opposition to SUT has swiftly given way to a general acceptance of the many advantages that disposables provide, including more flexibility and a smaller initial financial outlay. An increasing number of production facilities and manufacturing suites are constructed with disposable technology in an agile and flexible way. The primary aim of these plants is production for single use.

In addition to balancing media and single-use prices, these upstream technologies should account for processing timeframes in the overall production process timelines and the number of batches generated annually. Additionally, using SUT in smaller bioreactor applications could provide flexibility. A facility that has minimal limitations on changeover time and cleanliness verification can handle more lots and items.

Single-use technology has experienced significant evolution and continuous innovation in the last few years. Drug manufacturers have increased flexibility and capacity when single-use components are strategically used in a facility to enable quick configuration for numerous procedures and batch changes.

While equipment is SUT's primary focus, the structure and design of the building are also highly significant. Adding a modular building is becoming more common these days, particularly for businesses who want to retain some elements of a traditional facility. Two important qualities are the size and the convenience of use. A quicker launch of the production site is made possible by preconfigured configurations.

With SUT, you may easily develop a process at one manufacturing location and relocate it to another once the facility is operational. By connecting platform operations with single-use components, development times, effort, and time for equipment requirements, suitability, and parallel activities are reduced.

SUT providers are constantly thinking of new methods to enhance systems that currently exist, such as utilizing a single piece of equipment for several jobs. Among the examples are the Smart Flexware solutions from EMD Millipore. These systems demand less space and money because they are compatible with both chromatography and tangential flow filtration (TFF) techniques. Research contrasting SUT with stainless steel has allegedly demonstrated a minimum of 15% reduction in total expenses. The most recent advancements in single-use parts minimize COGS, increase process robustness, automate process management, and lower total costs.

Reliability of cross-contamination between batches is a top priority for regulatory organizations that produce biopharmaceuticals. Because it is impossible to rely on cleaning validation to ensure that minute quantities of contaminants from previous batches do not change the structure of proteins, the problem is far more serious than it is for chemical medications. Because of this, addressing the cGMP issue in the production of biological products is challenging. In addition, the increased demand has necessitated the use of quick, easy, and inexpensive production techniques.

Some of these problems have been fixed when comparing traditional stainless-steel systems to SUTs. Over the past 30 years, a method has been developed whereby top suppliers, like Pall, Sartorius, and Millipore, have taken the lead in producing disposables that are pre-sterilized and gamma-irradiated, eliminating the need for cleaning validation procedures.

The initial SUT components in this category were basic filters. These swiftly established themselves as the standard; at the moment, over 95% of the filters used in bioprocessing are disposable. After that, the focus shifted to other process components, which resulted in the creation of purification chromatography technologies and bioreactors. Two more process improvements that have allowed for relatively small-scale operations are high titers and process intensification (10,000 L stainless steel vs. 2,000 L single-use bioreactors). Because of its lower costs, smaller, more efficient facility, quicker batch turnaround, and removal of CIP and SIP, the SUT is today regarded as a significant advance in biopharmaceutical manufacturing.

Among other production phases in the biopharmaceutical manufacturing process, SUT components help with clone selection, cell banking, GMP production, formulation, fill-finish, and upstream and downstream process creation. Combining SUT with platform protocols allows for a quick transition from clone selection to GMP goods. The use of SUTs is growing, particularly in small-scale or clinical production. Until recently, single-use systems were unable to manage large batch quantities; however, TFF chromatography systems and other more modern technologies can.

While regulatory agencies do not require the development of single-use or disposable items, it is the responsibility of the manufacturer to ensure that cross-contamination limits are adhered to. When it takes a lot of effort and money to meet those requirements, the cost of single-use or disposable items becomes important. The FDA and EMEA strongly advise producers to develop settings that would keep pollutants out and verify the efficacy of cleanliness through validation techniques, as opposed to only cleaning goods. In order to create medications made from human and animal tissue, regulatory authorities' stance stiffened when virus contamination first surfaced in the 1970s. Many manufacturers stopped producing goods because they could not comply with the new rules. The transmissible spongiform encephalopathy outbreak added even more complexity, driving up the cost of producing biological drugs in cGMP-compliant facilities to unaffordable levels. On the other hand, the lack of regulatory guidance about the qualification requirements for these systems has been a significant issue with single-use technology.

It is evident that SUT offers benefits: it is safer, greener, more adaptable, and less costly (particularly when it comes to capital expenses). In the mainstream of manufacturing, there are still problems with the level of automation that can be accomplished with these components, scalability, operational costs, and material quality. The necessity for staff training to incorporate these elements into an established bioprocessing system, testing for extractable and leachable compounds, and reliance on supplier chains are further concerns.

While the EMA has approved a vaccine created using SUT, the FDA has not yet cleared a product developed using the method. There are currently a number of applications pending approval.

4.4.1 CONTAINERS AND MIXING SYSTEMS

Disposable or single-use bag systems are frequently utilized in place of containers with inflexible walls. This is because pharmaceutical products such as sterile intravenous solutions, blood, plasma, plasma expanders, and hyperalimentation solutions have historically been stored and dispensed using these types of bags. Typically, a single-layer film made of polyvinyl chloride or ethylene-vinyl acetate would be used in disposable bags to store blood (PVC). Single-use containers are widely utilized in biomanufacturing for a number of applications, such as cryopreservation bags, buffer and solution tank liners, mixing bags, microcarrier filter bags, and media storage (bottles, 2D, 3D, and two-ply and three-ply bioprocess bags). Common procedures involving mixing include dissolving buffer components, heating or chilling liquids, refolding solutions, scattering cell cultures in bioreactors, and culture media.

4.4.2 DRUMS, CONTAINERS, AND TANK LINERS

Simple, disposable bags called tank liners are used to line transportation systems and shipping containers. They are usually not gamma sterilized because they are used in open systems, such as the first preparation stage when making buffer solutions and culture medium. However, there are also tank liners that have already been steril-ized. Tank liners are less expensive than dedicated stainless steel or poly tanks and containers. The liner's only function inside the container is to provide mechanical support. When contour liners are used, conventional containers require less cleaning, validating, and sterilizing. Most importantly, because they are single-use, there is a lower possibility of cross-contamination with other products.

For smaller volumes, there are single-use, 50 mL–20L containers with an inte-grated handle, integrated hanging capabilities, and a needle-free sampling outlet. These are compatible with a sterile welder and are referred to as manifold system containers.

Most industry-standard cylindrical tanks with capacities ranging from 50 to 750L can be equipped with top or bottom draining, 2D or 3D lined cylindrical tanks. These tank liners are normally constructed in accordance with cGMP criteria in an ISO-classified cleanroom to minimize bioburden and other particle matter. Tank liners eliminate the need for pre- and post-cleaning, reducing cycle times. These are widely used for preparing buffers, hydrating media that is powdered, and creating various non-sterile solutions.

Connecting tank liners to commercially available overhead mixers is simple because most tank liners are open systems. However, tank liners should only be used with specific mixing systems that have a bottom-driven impeller. It is often better to utilize mixing methods without any mechanical parts inside the bag to reduce expenses, the chance of spinning devices injuring the bag, the bag grinding, or the stirrer inside the bag (either 2D or 3D). Better sterility is also provided by magneti-cally field stirring systems as opposed to magnetically connected ones.

Combining mixing systems with temperature sensors and load cells is another option. In addition, the tank liners may have provisions for pH testing, either single-use or reusable, and sample ports. The load cell, also known as the weight measurement, is the most crucial part. Even though most factories would use a floor scale, large-scale production requires installing load cells in the outer containers to prevent relocating the containers for weighing. Interestingly, the more costly systems include programming features that might make using the process analyti-cal technology (PAT) easier. However, by using the simplest and least expensive devices, the problems are negligible and can be resolved at the buffer and media preparation stages.

Many major equipment providers offer a complete line of mixing systems. While these can handle large volumes with reliability, a system can be created far more cheaply and easily with readily available components. Suppliers offer a range of choices for low-density polyethylene liners. Among the popular choices that cater to a range of industries include Sartorius, EMD Millipore's Mobius® Single-Use Mixing Systems, and Thermo Scientific's HyperformaTM line.

4.4.3   Two-Dimensional Pouches

2D bags are available in sterile, ready-to-use quantities ranging from 5 mL to 50L, ideal for smaller volumes before they become too big to manage. Media, buffer, clarified harvest, intermediate product, drug, and drug product can all be used using these bags. They are designed for transportation, filtration, sampling, and storage.

Additionally, these bags have connectors to other sterile single-use systems that are sterilely connected. It may occasionally be necessary to store powders in bags, including excipients, buffer salts, and API. These funnel-shaped bags are additive-free, antistatic, and equipped with large sanitary fittings or aseptic transfer systems.

4.4.4 PERSONALIZED TOTE BAGS

The 2D bags' larger-scale design flaw makes it more difficult to maintain their integrity, which causes handling and shipping issues. When 2D bags are completely filled, the weight of the fluid seeps through to the seams, potentially shattering the seals. The problem becomes more challenging when the 2D bags are rocked or shaken, as this puts extra strain on the seams.

When employing 3D bags as liners in hard-walled containers, integrity difficulties with 2D bags are eliminated; these bags are now available in a variety of sizes. Furthermore, the three-dimensional layout provides an additional space for the installation of ports with complex functionality. The 3D bags are made by fusing films together and come in cube, conical, or cylindrical shapes. The design of these containers is often determined by how they are stacked or positioned within other identically shaped containers, which allows the 3D bags to fit tightly. Numerous different solutions can be stored and transported in these 3D bags. They enable quick process adoption because they arrive sterile and ready to use right away.

Single-use bags are convenient for storing and transporting frozen products, from biological API delivery to cell culture as Working cell bank (WCB) for direct introduction into a bioreactor. Conversely, flexible bags are resistant to temperature changes; however, damage sustained during transit is often undetectable, thus a protective surface is required to reduce the danger.

Plastic disposable containers offer the best substitute for using disposable components because they don't need to be cleaned or validated. Low-density Polyethylene (PE) liners in a plastic container with a stiff wall and a standard mixer are the least expensive set of parts for making buffers and media. It is unnecessary to use more expensive specialized containers to transport these PE liners or more complex mixing methods.

4.4.5 ADVANTAGES

Using hybrid or single-use systems is a faster, more flexible, and less capital-intensive option. It is necessary to evaluate each option's costs and advantages in relation to production volume requirements, technological constraints, and infrastructural conditions. There are various advantages to using single-use production procedures over traditional stainless-steel equipment.

- Quicker time to market,
- Reduced capital: More batches, increased facility and equipment usage,
- Reduce or do away with cleaning and validation costs: The autoclave and SIP/CIP processes account for the majority of the 800,000 gallons of water

used daily by a biologic production unit. The upcoming generation of single-use gadgets wouldn't need these.

- Elimination of carryover,
- Increased flexibility for facilities with a variety of products, different batch sizes, and quicker turnaround times, as well as better cost adaptation to shifting scales and new modalities. When paired with modular facilities, SUT enables plug-and-play capabilities.
- Eliminate open processing and link unit operations to reduce the chance of cross-contamination. This makes it possible to think of multiple product processing or even step processing that happens simultaneously.

When assessing a single-use option for a particular process step, the cost-benefit analysis should include an evaluation of the possible effects on other process stages (e.g., previous and subsequent steps). Cost analysis should compare the fixed costs related to a stainless-steel process with the overall expenses of the production process. Perhaps the largest obstacle to the widespread acceptance of single-use products is the inability of manufacturers to deduct their large expenditures in fixed equipment and systems, which they built relatively recently (the 1970s and 1980s). Smaller companies, academic organizations, and contract enterprises are therefore the ones going through these changes. However, things will soon change drastically. Blockbuster recombinant medication patents are beginning to expire, giving smaller businesses the opportunity to compete on price. By posing a challenge to the high manufacturing costs that were deemed acceptable by major pharmaceutical corporations, the biosimilar industry should convince the industry to embrace the future of bioprocessing. There are environmental considerations to make.

If upstream and downstream processes are integrated with an innovative single-use strategy, a flexible, small-footprint facility can be achieved. In the long run, this helps in the production of affordable and efficient pharmaceuticals. a building made entirely of disposable, single-use parts. Numerous assessments indicate that the operating costs of a single-use facility are cheaper than those of a stainless-steel factory (Figure 4.1).

4.4.6 SINGLE-USE BIOREACTOR (SUBS)

With a rich history, the discipline of bioprocessing has produced a wide range of goods, most notably biopharmaceuticals, as well as novel techniques for biologics. The area was established many millennia ago. Cell culture needed two decades of trial and error, moving from a benching process at milligram sizes to industrial production at kilogram scales. Biopharmaceuticals are a contemporary phenomenon, produced on a huge scale in bioreactors made of stainless steel. These massive, 10,000–100,000 L capacity stirred-tank bioreactors are a mainstay of the biopharmaceutical sector and a testament to the status of mammalian cell culture technology.

Stainless steel bioreactors have been around for ages. Conventional bioreactor designs easily provide the required parts, which include a vessel large enough to house culture and media with adequate mixing and aeration. We have a wealth of

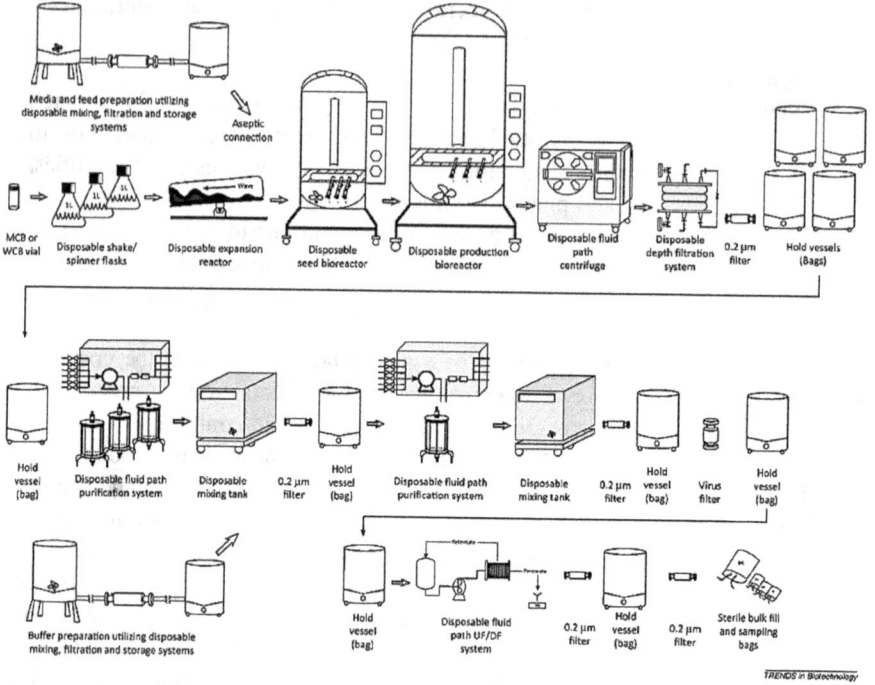

FIGURE 4.1 A biopharmaceutical manufacturing process built with single-use systems.

alternatives when it comes to bioreactor design today. These evolved when more biological drugs were produced in bioreactors, requiring the usage of various control features that weren't needed or required in other industries. Modification of conventional bioreactors was necessary to meet the increasing demands of these new engines of production, which included the manufacture of therapeutic proteins, vaccines, antibodies, and other products employing plant, animal, and viral cells. These new engines have advanced to the forefront of biological drug synthesis thanks to recombinant engineering. One notable recent modification to bioreactor design that reduces regulatory barriers in drug development is the use of single-use bioreactors to avoid cleaning validation difficulties. In addition to being widely used to provide medical supplies, disposable bioreactors are being used to study hundreds of novel chemicals.

Nearly all the recombinant medications on the market today were developed by big pharmaceutical corporations since the traditional bioreactor was the only accessible alternative some 40 years ago. The cost of the changeover protocols needed to be completed made it unfeasible to convert to another production method, even though their process would be less efficient.

A notable benefit of single-use bioreactors is their increased flexibility and substantially quicker changeover times. For example, the changeover time of a 200L bioreactor has been reduced to just 2–3 hours, compared to 24–48 hours for a stainless-steel reactor.

SUBS are made of Class VI plastic films, are gamma sterilized, and are discarded after use, even though their designs and purposes differ greatly. Additionally, they can be equipped with different attachments that allow for the recording of parameters linked to PAT, such as temperature monitoring, pH, dissolved oxygen (DO), OD, and media filtration. Using mechanical or hydraulic techniques, stirrers, paddles, shaking, and rocking the bags all combine to mix and aerate the contents of the bag as effectively as a conventional stainless-steel tank, often even more so.

SUBS have capacities ranging from milliliters to thousands of liters; they can be operated manually or entirely automatically; and their control systems can be as simple as a plastic bag or as complex as the priciest hard-walled bioreactors seen in traditional bioreactors. The market for disposable bioreactors is dynamic, with new developments emerging almost daily. Glass Petri dishes, T flasks, roller bottles, and glass flasks can be substituted with disposable hollow fiber systems, wave bioreactors, stirring 3D reactors, plastic plates, polypropylene, and Teflon bags for small-scale bacterial and yeast culturing.

Examples of stirring mechanisms include mechanical stirrers that are fastened to motors, magnetic stirrers that levitate without coming into touch with the motor, magnetic stirrers that rub off the surface from the bottom, and mechanical stirrers that are driven in from above. The most common motion is the rocking wave, which was created by Wave Bioreactor and is currently offered by a number of equipment manufacturers. The stationary bioreactor concept maintains the bag stationary, in contrast to the usual wave motion that requires switching out the plate. Rather, a flapper applies pressure on the edge of the disposable bag.

Three-dimensional single-use stirred tank reactor systems have shown to be a successful imitation of conventional stainless-steel reactors. The measurements, proportions, sparging systems, and mixing systems are similar to the conventional stainless-steel systems (reusable). The single-use bioreactor system consists of a sparger ring or microsparger, two axial flow three-blade segment impellers, or one axial flow three-blade segment and one radial flow six-blade segment impeller. The focused stirring technique ensures a homogeneous mixing of the bag. Each SUB is equipped with a temperature, mix, sparge, and vent monitor. Features for pH, harvest ports, liquid transfer, sampling, inoculation ports, and DO monitoring are included with the bioreactor bags (both reusable and single-use). SUBs allow plug-and-play setup and operation by standard sterile connections, and they interact readily with the most commonly used control systems in the industry. The SUBs reduce the need for cross-contamination risks, cleaning, and sterilization. Because of their wide volume range, these SUBs are suitable for large-scale cGMP manufacturing, clinical manufacturing, and process development (Figure 4.2).

Additionally, 2D single-use bioreactors like the CellBag that are specifically made for WAVE systems have been successfully used. Rock these bioreactor bags back and forth to stir them up. These bags are made from two-layer films that are fused together at the ends. The finished product is a flat chamber with either face- or end-welded apertures. Mostly used for the seed train stages, these WAVE bioreactors have capacity limitations and have trouble with large-scale agitation and aeration. Additionally, they take the place of the first disposable bioreactors, such as cell factories, roller bottles, and hollow fiber bioreactors. This is due to the fact that most

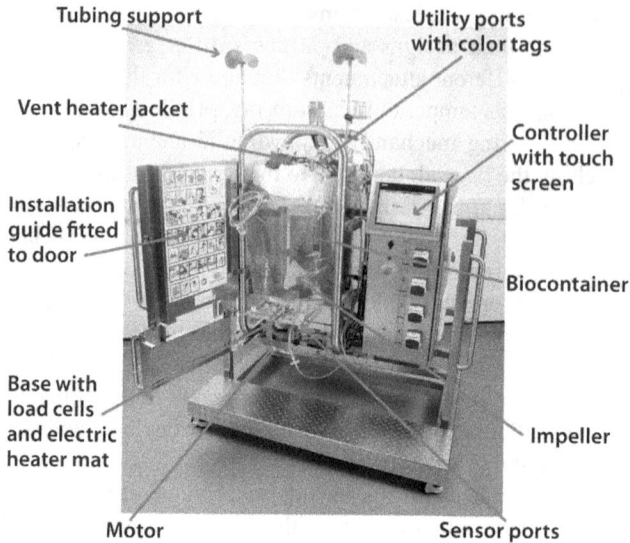

FIGURE 4.2 Single-use bioreactor. (https://bioprocessintl.com/2016/design-performance-single-use-stirred-tank-bioreactors/.)

animal and human cells proliferate in suspension without serum and that growing product titers are now causing cell culture bioreactor sizes to shrink.

The application of noninvasive optical sensor technologies to transparent animal cell culture containers has resulted in the creation of highly automated or tightly monitored and controlled disposable micro-bioreactor systems. This has made it easier to faithfully reproduce situations on a bigger scale and allowed early-stage process development to move from being completely unmonitored to fully specified and regulated.

The pharmaceutical industry's current desire for safe, individualized drugs is projected to fuel disposable bioreactor growth (such as functioning cancer cells, personalized antibodies, and immunological and tissue replacement therapies). When it comes to reaching optimal cell densities and product titers in the shortest amount of time, cell culture operators need to be willing to deviate from their tried-and-true method of using stirring devices. In addition to highly instrumented, scaled, wave-mixed, and stirred single-use bioreactors, shaken disposable bioreactors and novel techniques like the PBS or the BayShake are becoming more and more popular.

ThermoFisher, Cytiva Life Science (formerly GE Life Sciences), Sartorius, Eppendorf, and other bioreactor manufacturers have demonstrated how to effectively use SUBs for bacterial cultivation to enable high cell density mammalian culture.

4.4.7 Extra Components

According to the FDA Guidance for Industry (https://www.fda.gov/media/71012/download), PAT aims to promote innovation and efficiency in pharmaceutical research. PAT is a system that ensures the quality of the final product by designing, analyzing, and controlling manufacturing processes through timely measurement of critical quality and performance attributes of raw and in-process materials and processes (i.e., during processing). It is important to keep in mind that the word "analytical" in PAT encompasses a wide variety of integrated mathematical, microbiological, physical, chemical, and risk studies.

Single-use sensors, which are either integrated into the bioreactor or are part of the cover and are disposed of along with it, are required to meet certain process conditions. They provide a steady signal that allows one to always know how the cell culture is doing.

Since disposable bioreactors are a relatively new technology on the market, standard biosensors found in hard-walled systems were initially used to evaluate the bioreactor's output's temperature, conductivity, pH, DO, and osmolality. These probes must be autoclaved to guarantee sterilization before they are connected to penetration adapter fittings that are welded into bioreactor bags. Not surprisingly, this is a time-consuming and labor-intensive process that may compromise the integrity and sterility of single-use bioreactor bags. However, with advancements in SUB technology and technology in general, this has generally been dropped in favor of fully disposable sensors. Important process parameters, including cell density, UV absorbance, pH, DO, and pressure, are regularly monitored. Packages containing the traditional technologies for monitoring these parameters are usually not effective or compatible when integrated into single-use assemblies for a variety of reasons, such as cost, cross-contamination, inability to maintain a closed system, and system incompatibility with gamma irradiation. For these challenges, some of the measurements must be conducted offline.

It needs a deep understanding of the function and use of disposable sensors to get acceptability. The factors that determine their suitability include material properties, sensor manufacturing, process compatibility, performance requirements, control system integration, compatibility with pre-use treatments, and regulatory requirements.

Single-use solutions for process parameter monitoring can be even more cost-effective than tracking and maintaining traditional technologies, as they do not always preclude the use of traditional measurement technologies. They also eliminate the risk and expense associated with making process connections, as well as the need for equipment cleaning and small-part autoclaving. A sanitary, autoclavable pressure transducer that is authorized for a certain number of autoclave cycles and needs to be recalibrated may be less expensive to operate than a single-use pressure sensor.

There are two applications for disposable sensors: in situ, where the sensors are in contact with the liquid, and ex-situ, where the sensors are removed from the medium either by a sterile, disposable sample removal tool or by optical means (online). Single-use sensors should be inexpensive, trustworthy, and able to be sanitized or supplied already sterilized if they come into contact with media. Better designs combine inexpensive sensing components inside a disposable bioreactor with reusable (and more costly) analytical equipment outside the reactor. Cheap, one-time sensors can also be put on transistors and placed in the headspace, input, outflow, or culturing broth for liquid-phase analysis (temperature, pH, and pO_2). Another alternative for these would be optical sensors, which allow for covert observation through a clear glass.

4.4.8 Measurements with Optics

The effect of electromagnetic waves on molecules is the principle underlying the operation of optical sensors. It is an entirely non-invasive method that can provide continuous findings for numerous parameters at the same time. Because the bioreactors have a clear window, using them is rather easy. The detector component of the system can be physically segregated, which allows the online or in situ usage of optical sensors with expensive analytical equipment.

Fluorescence sensors can be enhanced for nicotinamide adenine dinucleotide phosphate (NADH) readings and are used to differentiate between aerobic and anaerobic metabolism (NADPH). Additionally, biomass is estimated using them. The two-dimensional process of fluorometry enables the simultaneous detection of many analytes, such as proteins, vitamins, coenzymes, biomass, glucose, and metabolites including ethanol, adenosine-5′-triphosphate, and pyruvate, by scanning a range of excitation and emission wavelengths. Thus, the upstream process can be characterized using fluorometry. The greatest outcomes are typically obtained by mounting a fiber-optic lamp on the bioreactor and shining it through a glass window. One example of this is the fluorometers in the BioView system (www.bioview.com). A multichannel fluorescence detection tool, the BioView sensor finds utility in biotechnology, food production, pharmaceutical, and environmental monitoring applications. It can determine specific chemicals, the state of microorganisms, and the chemical environment in which they live without modifying the sample. The BioView system measures fluorescence in real time online throughout the procedure. The likelihood of contamination is reduced when interference with the sample is eliminated. However, the complexity of the spectra of multiple components requires high-level resolution programming.

Many different types of metabolic products in a bioreactor can be easily identified with IR spectroscopy. However, a water-absorbed infrared beam can only be NIR or SIR for biomass analysis when used in transmission mode. ATR-IR probes for bioreactors and NIR transmission probes are commercially available solutions. These are connected via silver halide fibers or radio frequency links.

Besides infrared and fluorescent technologies, optical methods based on photoluminescence, reflection, and absorption are also used. As with fluorescence detectors, they can use these chemosensors in situ or online by attaching the optical electrodes, or optodes, using glass fibers that leave the measuring device outside the bioreactor.

A fluorescent dye (metal complexes) needs to be immobilized and attached to one end of an optical fiber in order to detect oxygen. Molecular oxygen quenches fluorescence in oxygen sensors to enable their operation. The opposing end of the fiber is interfaced with an excitation light source. The duration and intensity of the fluorescence are influenced by the oxygen level of the surrounding air. After the bioreactor releases its fluorescence light, it is collected and sent outside for examination. Compared to traditional platinum probe electrodes, these electrodes are more efficient at detecting oxygen because they can operate in both liquid and gas phases. One noninvasive oxygen sensor that monitors the partial pressure of both gaseous and dissolved oxygen is called PreSens (www.presens.de). Disposables and glasses are used in conjunction with these sensor sites. The sensor dots are affixed to the inside surface of the glass or clear plastic material. Therefore, the oxygen concentration can be externally and non-destructively measured via the vessel wall. A wide selection of coatings with different concentration ranges are available. Depending on flow rate and gas phase oxygen measurement, it offers real-time online monitoring of DO concentrations between 1 ppb and 45 ppm. These are autoclavable.

Ocean Optics is selling the first small spectrometer in the world with several gas phases, pH, and oxygen sensors (www.oceanoptics.com).

Fiber-optic pH measurements can be performed using indicators based on absorbance or fluorescence. pH sensors work by absorption or fluorescence. Fluorescein and derivatives of 8-hydroxyl,3,6-pyrene trisulfonic acid are the most often used dyes for fluorescence, whereas phenol red and cresol red are used to assess absorption type. Fluorescent dyes cannot be employed for large-scalepH measurements due to their sensitivity to ionic strength (more than three units).

The fundamental concept of carbon dioxide sensors is to measure the pH of a carbonate buffer that is protected from CO_2 by a membrane. Quaternary ammonium hydroxide reacts faster than the sensors because of its shorter reaction time.

Fluorescence-based sensors are attractive because they simplify the creation of low-cost, portable devices that may be rapidly assembled outside of a laboratory. These measurements are not affected by changes in the instrument or variations in the dye concentration, leaching, or photobleaching of the fluorophore, in contrast to unreferenced fluorescence intensity measurements. The performance of the sensor system exhibits high levels of repeatability, reversibility, and stability.

4.4.8.1 Biomass Sensors

Another instrument that can be used to collect information on biomass concentration is a turbidity sensor. Usually, these sensors work using the scattered light theory. Most turbidity sensors have the limitation that the correlation is only linear at low particle concentrations. However, sensors using 180° backscattering light also exhibit linear properties for high particle concentrations. For the intended infrared wavelength, disposable reactors need a translucent window. The S3 Mini-Remote Futura line of biomass detectors (www.applikonbio.com) is operated by sensors located inside disposable bioreactors. This system features an extremely lightweight pre-amplifier for connecting to the ABER disposable probe (https://www.bioprocess-eng.co.uk/product/aber-futura-pico/).

4.4.8.2 Electrochemical Sensors

Electrochemical sensors include voltammetric, conductometric, and potentiometric sensors. Chemically sensitive field-effect transistors (ChemFETs) and thick- and thin-film sensors have prospective use as potentiometric disposable sensors in bioprocess control due to their large-scale, low-cost manufacturing.

Many pH monitors rely on amperometry methods, which are unstable or prone to wander and require constant calibration. Most amperometry sensor setups are based on the pH-dependent selectivity of membranes or films on the electrode surface.

While capacitance sensors provide accurate information about the mass of live cells, turbidity sensors detect the concentration of biomass overall. Electrical capacitance and conductance are frequently used to describe the electrical properties of cells in an alternating electrical field. The electrical impedance is highly dependent on the integrity of the cell membrane in order to estimate only live cells. The Biodis Series is provided by Hamilton (https://www.hamiltoncompany.com) and Aber for tracking sustainable biomass in disposable applications (www.aberinstruments.com). as well as an integrated Eppendorf version (www.eppendorf.com).

4.4.8.3   Measurements of Pressure

Pressure is an important process parameter that is frequently observed in various bioprocess unit operations, including filtering and chromatography. A traditional stainless-steel pressure gauge can be used in conjunction with a single-use experimental setup; however, the pressure gauge must be cleaned separately. Additionally, there can be problems connecting the sensor to the single-use component that was previously subjected to gamma radiation.

Many bioprocess unit operations are largely controlled by pressure or there are significant safety issues. Conventional stainless-steel reactors regulate and monitor pressure because it impacts mass transfer and contributes to the reactor's cleanliness. A situation with a lot of pressure might also be dangerous. The vent filter of a bioreactor may quickly clog, exposing the operators to unprocessed bulk and the contents of the reactor when bags break.

Another area where pressure monitoring is critical to process effectiveness is the depth and sterile filtering procedure. The two primary markers of a filter's capacity are either pressure increases or flow degradation. However, adding reusable conventional pressure transducers to a process train defeats the purpose of a single-use process configuration. Depending on the process application, a typical device's product contact surface needs to be either sterilized or sanitized using moist heat.

Steam in place (SIP), where steam is applied only to the product contact surface, and even autoclavable devices, where steam is applied to the entire device, are both compatible with conventional devices. Many single-use process components are incompatible with wet heat sterilization temperatures; thus, the stainless-steel device might need to be sterilized separately and connected to a pre-sterilized single-use assembly in a less-than-ideal way.

Early-stage clinical manufacturing and development applications can easily replace product contact components thanks to single-use pressure sensing. For example, PendoTECH (www.pendotech.com) sells single-use assemblies with flexible tubing serving as the fluid channel for pressure sensors that are meant to make pressure measurement easier. These single-use pressure sensors' fluid path materials are gamma compatible and meet EMEA 410 Rev 2 and USP Class VI requirements (up to 50 KGy).

The USP Class VI accreditation is ideally suited for medical applications because it is believed to be the harshest. It includes the three in vivo biological reactivity tests mentioned below, which are frequently performed on mice or rabbits to mimic human use:

The degree of toxicity and irritation that results from a drug being injected topically, breathed, swallowed, or coming into touch with the skin is assessed using the Acute Systemic Toxicity (Systemic Injection) test.

Intradermal test: Evaluates the sample's localized toxicity and irritation when it comes into contact with living subcutaneous tissue (specifically, the tissue that the medical device is intended to contact).

The implantation test assesses the irritability, toxicity, and risk of infection of a chemical after it is injected intramuscularly into a test animal over a number of days.

The chemical needs to have extremely low toxicity and pass all three tests. Additionally, it will be evaluated at different temperatures for pre-arranged periods of time. USP Class VI materials typically ensure a high-quality level and greater acceptance by the FDA and USDA since they are believed to greatly reduce the risk of patient injury from a hazardous material response.

However, USP Class VI Testing is only one standard for biocompatibility. ISO-10993 is a stricter standard for the biological inspection of medical equipment. However, some biocompatibility requirements for medical equipment could be higher than those tested in USP Class VI.

ISO-10993 uses both systemic toxicity testing and intracutaneous reactivity testing. However, it also includes more thorough testing for hemocompatibility, cytotoxicity, genotoxicity, chronic toxicity, and systemic toxicity. Medical devices that are going to be permanently or semi-permanently implanted into a patient are primarily required to go through the various ISO-10993 testing standards. Therefore, for devices that are not intended for implant or that will have minimal patient interaction, ISO-10993 testing might be more stringent than necessary.

Installing a sensor on a vent line allows one to measure the headspace pressure in a single-use bioreactor. Although the sensors are authorized for use up to 75 psi, the core sensor is accurate in the low-pressure range required for a single-use bioreactor.

4.4.9 Sampling

Sampling is a standard method in manufacturing to measure in-process parameters like pH, DO, OD, pCO_2, etc. to guarantee compliance. Most single-use systems have one or more integrated sample lines that are partially equipped with special sampling manifolds, valves, or systems. The Clave connector is a popular single-use sample valve that is also used in intravascular catheters for medical applications; it may be purchased from ICU-Medical (www.icumed.com). It facilitates the use of a Luer-Lok syringe for sample collection. The sample is only in contact with the aseptic inner components of the valve thanks to its dynamic seal, which also makes sure that it is not taken until the syringe is connected. However, the sterility of the extracted samples is lost.

Manifolds equipped with flasks, syringes, or sampling bags are appropriate for sampling aseptic samples in single-use systems. These manifolds can be connected to the systems by aseptic connectors or tube welding. Repeated sampling for quality control over a predetermined period of time is made possible by sampling manifolds. The main property of a manifold is the reduction in the number of operations needed in a process. Preassembled, sterilized, and sent ready for process use are the manifold systems. Filling several bags is made possible with just one connection.

Sampling is also done with manifold systems, where sample containers are arranged in parallel within the manifold; the last container is used as a waste container. The first flow and the succeeding sample are directed to the appropriate containers using tube clamps and Y-, T-, or X-hose barbs. Of course, SIP connections can also be used to link manifold systems to conventional stainless-steel processing machinery.

To obtain a sample devoid of organisms, a bioreactor can be continually sampled using a peristaltic pump and sterile filter. A needleless syringe and a presterilized sampling container that can be attached to the bag bioreactor's sampling module are both usable. After a sample is injected into the container and these sampling containers are taken out of the assembly, the tube is heat-sealed. In certain sampling systems, to prevent the sample from going back into the reactor, a presterilized Leuer connection with a one-way valve is connected. The sample is removed from the reactor using a syringe and placed via a sample line into a reservoir. For example, Millipore (https://www.sigmaaldrich.com) and Cellexus Biosystems (https://cellexus.com) use this tactic. The Cellexus system that is attached to the sample line has the capacity to hold up to six sealed sample pouches. The pouches can then be filled with the reservoir sample and mechanically sealed to produce sterile, sealed samples. Bioreactor manufacturers and producers provide a range of customizable sample manifolds.

The unique Millipore system is made up of several flexible conduits that are connected to flexible, single-use sampling containers that may be opened and closed independently for samples. It also comes with a port insert that is compatible with several ports on the bioreactor side. The sample limit is the number of conduits that are available in each module.

These sampling techniques allow for aseptic sampling; nevertheless, each module has restrictions regarding sample count and automation. Furthermore, even though these methods help produce high-quality validation data, there is always a chance of contamination because the bioreactor is breached every time a sample is retrieved. Alternative strategies that do not involve talking to the media must be developed.

4.4.10   CONNECTORS

The complexity of bioprocessing makes it difficult to create systems that are flawlessly designed. All connections, tubing, and equipment must be connected at separate points during the procedure to lower the risk of contamination, and sampling must be done in a sterile setting. Connections and lines were the first areas where single-use parts were employed since they were difficult to clean. Unlike rigid pipe, which can be costly and time-consuming to clean and verify, flexible tubing used in single-use transfer lines only needs to be done once. Because of this, manufacturers can quickly adapt their production procedures or transition to a new product. When the requirements for the processes change depending on the drug being produced, this is a huge benefit for multiple manufacturing sites. Innovative manufacturers are using single-use tube assemblies in bioprocesses more and more, from seed trains to final fill applications. Additional cost reductions result from lower labor, chemical, water, and energy requirements for cleaning and validation.

Steam is available for clean-in-place(CIP)/SIP operations, which is the primary reason SIP systems are used in hard-walled systems. Even then, there is still a possibility of contamination. Since the biomedical industry has produced a significant amount of the SUT needed in various applications, the device industry has consistently outperformed regulations. Regulators can request detailed information from manufacturers on their devices, and biocompatibility issues have long been resolved. Because of the intricacy of the manufacturing process, it is rare that a user will request a custom device; however, the range of alternatives available today is adequate to adapt any system that would employ an off-the-shelf item. It still emphasizes the value of off-the-shelf goods above custom creations. Tube connectors and sealers are a more recent innovation, as single-use bags for mixing and bioreactors have become more and more popular. Still, a limited number of vendors are available, the majority of them being Cytiva LifeSciences Sartorius-Stedim. The alternative option is to use expensive aseptic connectors, even if the cost of this equipment is still high. If a good selection of aseptic connections is available, they should generally be used instead of tube connectors since it is always possible to employ heat-activated systems to make a bad connection and because aseptic connectors let you connect tubes that might not be thermolabile.

In contemporary bioprocessing facilities, the inoculum is scaled up from a few million cells in several milliliters of culture to production volumes of hundreds of liters. Aseptic transfers are required at every stage of the seed train in this procedure. In traditional bioprocessing facilities, the process of scaling up is accomplished through the utilization of a particular series of stainless-steel bioreactors connected by stiff tubing and valves. In order to prevent contamination between production runs, a CIP system is included in every bioreactor, vessel, and pipeline in these systems. Both CIP and SIP systems require extensive validation testing, and additional validation problems could result from the pipes and valves inside these systems.

Thanks to developments in SUT, bioprocess engineers may now replace the majority of fixed pipe networks and storage tanks with single-use storage systems and tubing assemblies. Single-use components eliminate the need for pricey containers, valves, and sanitary pipe assemblies, which reduces maintenance and capital expenses. Additionally, they remove many components' need for CIP approval.

Single-use media storage systems are typically utilized with capacities ranging from 20 to 2,500 L. Media storage systems are prepared for delivery to the bioprocess facility by means of gamma irradiation. These systems often have built-in connectors, sampling devices, and filters. Operators can establish sterile connections between these presterilized single-use systems bioreactors for the aseptic transfer of media, cells, and any other liquid additions by employing single-use digital-to-analog connectors (DACs) or even tube welders and sealers with appropriate tubing. The DACs are also suitable for downstream applications. These aseptic connectors may be useful in applications where high flow and high pressure are required.

In a similar manner, the inoculum is moved between bioreactors by means of a peristaltic pump or headspace pressure, both of which require the use of specially made, pre-sterilized single-use tubing assemblies. Aseptic couplings on flexible tubing are used as transfer lines between each reactor in the process. These transfer lines reduce the number of reusable valves required for transfers and eliminate trouble spots for CIP and SIP validation. A single-use SIP connector can be used to terminate each presterilized transfer line, reducing capital costs while preserving the same degree of sterility assurance as conventional fixed pipes.

Liquids may need to be transferred from a higher ISO environment to a lower ISO environment in specific circumstances. A conduit with greater pressure in the cleaner room can be installed in the walls separating the two areas to make sure that this does not cause cross-contamination. A pre-sterilized tube is inserted from the lower ISO class side to the higher ISO class side of the vessels using a peristaltic pump to transfer liquid between them. The tube is moved into the higher ISO class region and disposed of after the transfer is finished. This method allows upstream and downstream areas to be connected without incurring the risk of contaminating another area with a lower ISO class or a downstream area.

4.4.11 TUBING

Flexible tubes are necessary for all single-use systems, but they are governed by the same safety concerns as the leachable and extractable materials covered in the preceding chapter. A few of the characteristics of flexible tubing that need to be assessed are its flexibility, operating temperature range, chemical resistance, color, density, shore hardness, flexibility, elasticity, surface smoothness, mechanical stability, abrasion resistance, gas permeability, visible and ultraviolet (UV) light sensitivity, layer composition, weldability, sealability, and sterilizability by gamma radiation or in an autoclave.

Each tube used in bioprocessing conforms to USP Class VI classification, FDA 21 CFR 177.2600, and EP 3A Sanitary Standard. These are classified as bulk drugs for cGMP manufacturing.

4.4.12 PUMPS

By creating differential or hydrostatic pressure, pumps are utilized to move fluids; the highest pressure that may be applied depends on the bioprocess component that is least resistant to the pressure. Some unit operations, like harvesting, TFF, and chromatography, need the molecule to be very sensitive to changes in pumping. The pulsing could damage the pump's internal parts or have an impact on the fluid being pumped. The pump must have the following characteristics in order to be suitable for the use for which it is intended.

- low exposure with respect to surface area and volume
- minimum levels of leachable and extractable
- controlled flow and pressure
- minimal shear and pulsation
- Absence of mechanical spalling or contact material shedding
- Self-priming
- Not a build-up of heat
- Sterility
- increased efficacy in volume

Permanent stainless-steel process lines are complex, expensive to build, and require a lot of cleaning and validation. Because they use mechanical seals that can't maintain sterility or a consistent flow, some pumps aren't as good for handling biologics.

These days, peristaltic, syringe, and diaphragm pumps offer single-use pumping solutions. Single-use positive displacement quaternary diaphragm pumps are among the best options for bioprocessing applications. Although these volume displacement pumps are easy to use and keep the substance out of reach, they may overstress the tubing, especially if operations are prolonged. Particles generated by tension-induced erosion of the tube may contaminate the fluids being passed through. By supplying low pressure and handling biological substances gently, peristaltic pumps protect them from shear stress. However, biological products could be harmed by the quick flow through microscopic holes created by a piston pump's valve system. Even valve-less piston pumps use high shear factors and pressures, which could be detrimental to biological products.

High-end peristaltic dispensing pumps now function better, thanks to improved pulsation-free pump heads, precise drive motors, and modern calibration algorithms. They are extremely accurate in terms of microliter fill volumes. Since single-use tubing is the only part in contact with the substance, it prevents cross-contamination and the need for cleaning in peristaltic pumps. Peristaltic pumps with single-use tubing offer far easier cleaning validation processes than piston pumps. On the other hand, peristaltic pumps may have problems with viscous products. The pumps lose accuracy while handling pressures higher than about 1.3 bar and are unable to handle products with viscosities more than 100 cP. Many developments in pumps intended for downstream processing, including high-performance liquid chromatography (HPLC), TFF, and virus filtration (VF) applications (e.g., Quantum; https://www.watson-marlow.com/us-en/range/watson-marlow/single-use-pumps/quantum/), have made it possible to achieve high process yields across the pressure range. In addition to being composed of bags rather than stainless steel containers, single-use pumps frequently call for specific agitators, couplings, valves, and single-use tubing. The single-use components eliminate the need for extensive validation and reduce cleaning costs. Plug-and-play options are included with TFF applications. These pumps increase the downstream process's production by causing ultra-low shear and supplying a steady flow across the required pressure range.

A diaphragm pump is a kind of positive displacement pump that uses suitable non-return check valves in combination with the reciprocating action of a Teflon, rubber, or thermoplastic diaphragm to pump a fluid. Reciprocating connecting plates provide the power for sequential quaternary diaphragm pumps. All other liquid biologics and thick liquids are easily handled by these pumps. Some pumps can also operate with minimum shear, pulsation, and heat buildup as self-priming, dry runs, and continuous flow devices.

4.4.13   TUBE WELDERS AND SEALERS

When employing a thermoplastic tube, welding offers an easy, reasonably priced, and very safe method. Examples of thermoplastic tubes are Bioprene, PharMed, and C-Flex. The two thermoplastic tubes must have the same end-cap, be aseptic, and have the same outer and inner diameters. The tubes are placed opposite and parallel to one another, and a heated blade is used to cut through and seal each tube at the same time. Preheating the blade is required to get it up to welding temperature as well as to clean and dehydrogenize it before welding. Dehydrogenation typically occurs in

3 seconds at 320°C or 30 seconds at 250°C. After cutting, all of the tubes connected to the aseptic systems are pushed up against one another until their ends are precisely opposite to one another on either side of the blade. A welding cycle can take 1–4 minutes, depending on the material and tube diameter. The main welding systems currently available on the market are the Sterile Tube Fuser (GE Healthcare), BioWelder (Sartorius-Stedim), Aseptic Sterile Welder 3,960 (SEBRA, www.Sebra.com), TSCD (Terumo, www.terumotransfusion.com), and SCD 11B. (Terumo). Sartorius-Stedim and GE Healthcare have the most installations in the bioprocessing industry (Terumo mostly offers equipment to the blood transfusion industry).

After disconnecting an aseptic connection, the ends can be sealed with a laminar hood or tube sealers, like those provided by PDC (www.pdcbiz.com), Saint-Gobain (www.Saint-Gobain.com), Sartorius-Stedim (www.sartorius-stedim.com), GE Healthcare (www.GE Lifesciences. com), Terumo (www.terumotransfusion.com), and SEBRA (www.sebra.com). Most of these sealers can seal tubes that range in size from 0.25 to around 1.5 and can complete the process in 1–4 minutes. While not all tube sealing techniques include radio waves or electrical heating sources, most do. It is not necessary to have a laminar flow cover for these tasks. Using a crimper twice and cutting the tube in between the crimps is usually the least expensive method.

4.5   WORKING DOWNSTREAM

Using single-use technology offers a compelling way to reduce downtime between batches, relieves the additional burden of cleaning, validates these procedures, and, most importantly, reduces the risk of contamination between batches. Single-use solutions also facilitate easy transitions between product lines in a multiproduct operation. SUTs have developed alongside downstream processes such as columns, different disposable hardware systems, and one-time-use flow paths since they have shown to be an efficient upstream solution.

Large-scale commercial manufacturing can be facilitated by single-use liquid chromatography systems, such as the ÄKTA ready XL chromatography systems with disposable flow pathways and prepacked columns, which can easily meet the capacity requirements of high-titer single-use 2,000-L upstream processes. It has been shown that these solutions are very beneficial for both technology transfer and process scale-up operations.

Encouraging therapeutic drugs to be cost-effective is becoming more and more important. Reducing the overall cost of manufacturing and investment requires the employment of continuous manufacturing (CM) operations and single-use solutions.

The employment of single-use components in downstream bioprocessing has changed over time, with sporadic innovative peaks. The initial items utilized were buffer bags and standard flow filtration apparatus, such as guard filters for chromatographic columns and virus filtering. But over time, more complex concepts have been put forth, like chromatography devices intended for single use and downstream processing tangential flow filtration. The industry consensus presently is that some downstream processing aspects will stay traditional, even while many upstream operations can be transformed into totally single-use systems. This claim is supported by

the arguments that it will always be too costly to discard resins and columns, and it will be difficult to discover a suitable single-use substitute for large-scale columns. However, history shows that only 15 years ago, these were the exact same arguments used to oppose the conversion of bioreactors to single-use equipment. Nowadays, the field of downstream processing is developing more quickly than that of upstream processing; membrane adsorbs have been proposed as a practical solution for large-scale antibody purification recently. When compared to conventional resins, these membranes are far less expensive.

4.5.1 CELL COLLECTION

A substitute for conventional centrifugation in the collection of cells and removal of waste is filtration. Systems for single-use filtering are available and offer scalability and operational flexibility. Benefits include the ease of scaling up and the availability of pre-sterilized filter capsules that are easily integrated into production processes. Even though centrifugation or lenticular filtration are typically used to complete this stage, the depth filter systems (like Millipore's POD Filtration) offered the first readily available alternative in single-use lenticular filters, combining two distinct separation technologies in an adsorptive depth filter to improve filter capacity and retention while condensing multiple filtration steps into one efficient operation. Depth filters use a porous filtration medium to retain particles throughout the medium instead of just on the surface. Depth filters are made of fibers that are dispersed across a substrate to produce a mesh. With the help of a binder, specific additives such as activated carbon, ceramic fibers, and others like materials are inserted to help create the filter. Retentive filters concentrate the filtered material on the surface, whereas depth filters retain particles based on adsorption effects and sieving by using their entire depth. These filters are widely used when the fluid to be filtered contains a high load of particles since they can hold a bigger quantity of particles before getting clogged than other types of filters.

Scale-up is achieved by inserting multiple pods into a holder; configurations accommodate 1–5 or 5–30 pods, depending on the requirement. Additional single-use depth filter forms include Millipore's Clarisolve, DOHC, and XOHC adsorptive depth filter for primary and secondary clarifying; the encapsulated Zeta Plus from Cuno; the L-Drum from Sartorius-Stedim; and the Stax-System from Pall Life Science. These filters allow for efficient cell clearing by reducing cell biomass, HCP, and host DNA while also removing most of the cell debris to produce a straightforward load on the chromatographic column.

The amount of colloid in the bioreactor offload and the upstream centrifuge's capacity to eliminate cell debris determine how well depth filters perform. When operating at a steady flow of 100–200 L/min, depth filters can run at up to 150 L of feed per m2 of filter, depending on the composition of the feed stream (m2 h). The Millipore Millistak+ Pod system has a maximum 33 m2 filter area capacity, which results in a batch capacity of 3–5,000 L. A larger 55 m2 filter area is possible, thanks to the Millipore Mobius FlexReady process equipment. Holding tanks with the appropriate volume can be lined with single-use PE liners because large amounts of buffers are required for the cleaning of these filters.

When processing large amounts of clarified harvest, crossflow filtration can be utilized to reduce the volume required for additional purification; however, debris buildup lengthens the filtration time. Using a single-use filter prevents cross-contamination even if it is not a sterile operation.

It is advised to process different recombinant proteins and vaccines using kSep® or other single-use continuous centrifugation equipment. Centrifugal force and feed flow combine to produce force in the kSep, a closed constant centrifuge. The continuous, low-shear operation of this technology permits efficient processing without sacrificing recovery. Each method has advantages and disadvantages, so it's best to experiment with them all and choose the method that works best for a particular strategy and type of cell. The above single-solution performance is influenced by the USP performance, cell density, vitality, and quantity of cell debris in the bioreactor broth.

4.5.2 PURIFICATION

To capturing and polishing, a resin (stationary phase) composed of porous beads made of a polysaccharide, mineral, or synthetic matrix connected to certain functional groups via a variety of separative principles is loaded into a steel column. The protein combination is injected into the column gradually along with other ingredients. Once the protein is bound to the resin and rinsed with the appropriate pH and electrolyte solutions, the target protein in the mixture is separated. The resin is cleaned and sanitized in order to get it ready for repeated use—dozens or even hundreds of cycles.

To reduce the time required to load resin and run a column, several vendors now provide columns for use in AKTA machines, such as GE's ReadyToProcess systems. In addition to a large selection of resins, GE also provides custom resins. High-performance bioprocessing columns, prepackaged, prequalified, and presanitized are what these are. Cross-contamination is prevented by the use of single-use or single-use flow pathways and ReadyToProcess columns. With its hygienic design, the ÄKTA ready system is ideal for usage in cGMP-regulated settings. Enhanced economy and productivity are made possible by the straightforward processes and short turnaround times between batches of ÄKTA ready items. Additional prepackaged columns such as the ReadyToProcess available are Opus (Repligen), GoPure, and (Life Technologies).

The AKTA system offers the same performance level as traditional processing columns like AxiChromTM and BPGTM since it is built for easy scaling. These are now offered in four distinct sizes—1, 2.5, 10, and 20 L—and are compatible with a variety of BioProcessTM medium. Their purpose is to purify biopharmaceuticals in preparation for clinical phase I and II investigations. They can also be utilized for preclinical research and full-scale manufacturing, depending on the size of the activities. The columns can be used to separate different molecules such as proteins, endotoxins, DNA, plasmids, vaccinations, and viruses in a variety of chromatographic applications.

To reduce the need for cleaning and validation, single-use chromatography solutions, like the AKTA XL systems, are available with prepacked columns, plug-and-play

TABLE 4.2
Various Membrane and Ligand Types

Membrane Type	Description	Ligand	Pore Size (μm)
Sulfonic acid (S)	Strong acidic cation exchanger	$R\text{-}CH_2\text{-}SO_3\text{---}$	>3
Quaternary ammonium (Q)	Strong basic anion exchanger	$R\text{-}CH_2\text{-}N\text{+}(CH_3)_3$	>3
Carboxylic acid(C)	Weak acidic cation exchanger	$R\text{-}COO\text{-}$	>3
Diethylamine (D)	Weak basic anion exchanger	$R\text{-}CH_2\text{-}N(C_2H_5)_2$	>3
Phenyl	Hydrophobic interaction (HIC)	Phenyl	>3
IDA	Metal chelate	Iminodiacetic acid	>3
Protein A	Affinity	Protein A	0.45
Epoxy-activated	Coupling	Epoxy group	0.45
Aldehyde-activated	Coupling	Aldehyde group	0.45

Source: Sartorius-Stedim.

chromatography columns, membranes, and single-use flow pathways in addition to presterilized filters and tubing. Chromatography systems designed for production and process scale-up that are ready for ÄKTA. uses single-use, ready-to-use flow routes that do not require cleaning or validation in between batches or goods.

Protein purification from complicated mixtures is a crucial step in the development and manufacturing of pharmaceuticals. However, particulate-matricule chromatography calls for drawn-out steps and long separation durations.

There are numerous ligands available, such as (Table 4.2).

One particular benefit of employing membrane adsorbers in the production of monoclonal antibodies is the elimination of impurities with large molecular weight, such as viruses and DNA. Since these compounds do not easily permeate conventional resins, significantly larger columns are necessary for the majority of polishing procedures that rely on column chromatography. Because of these hydrodynamic advantages, membrane adsorbers may be operated at substantially higher flow rates than columns, thereby lowering buffer consumption and cutting the processing time down to a factor of 100. Membrane adsorbers with commercial application include Mustang® (Pall), Sartobind® (Sartorius), Chromasorb® (Millipore), and Adsept® (Natrix). These membranes are frequently employed in flow-through mode to remove endotoxins and other contaminants associated with processes, such as DNA.

The Accelerated Seamless Antibody Purification method, which is based on AKTA periodic counter-current chromatography (PCC) Protein-A, mixed-mode, and anion exchange resin columns that are cycled simultaneously, is a single-use, continuous mAb downstream process. These systems combine flexibility, convenience of use, and greater capacity with the benefits of both single-use and continuous processing in a single application.

A robust supply chain is essential to consider when choosing single-use consumables. Maintaining regulatory compliance by making sure the appropriate paperwork and testing are done for extractable and leachable materials.

Single-use systems offer a great deal of flexibility in handling many items in a facility; faster product releases are achieved due to the short turnaround times between batches or products.

4.5.3 VIRUS ELIMINATION

All biotechnology products made from human or animal cell lines are susceptible to virus contamination. A product's therapeutic outcomes may be significantly affected if it contains endogenous viruses from cell banks or accidental viruses from staff members. Licensed biological goods are guaranteed to be virus-free, thanks to three complementing methods:

- comprehensive examination for viral contamination of the cell line and all source components,
- evaluating the downstream processing's ability to remove contagious viruses, and
- Examining the product at the proper stages to check for viral contamination.

There is a mix of size exclusion, adsorption, and inactivation techniques available. The FDA demands proof of viral clearance using two different techniques. Solvent and detergent, chemical treatments, low pH, and microwave heating are a few examples of inactivation techniques. Adsorption techniques make use of chromatography, while mechanical or molecular size exclusion techniques employ tangential flow and normal (forward) flow filtration techniques.

To eradicate viruses, ion exchange and Protein A chromatography are frequently employed, and significant research has been carried out in association with the FDA. However, the onus of demonstrating the appropriateness of any given approach continues to rest with the creator. For many years, membrane filtration has been utilized in mAb procedures to remove viruses. Some of the more recent single-use solutions for viral clearance include hollow-fiber membrane cartridges and even surface-modified, hydrophilic membranes with high void volume and minimum fouling that can reduce viral titers significantly. Adsorptive filters can be employed in conjunction with the viral filtration stage at the conclusion of the purifying procedure. Viral filtration efficiency is increased by these filters, which combine the concepts of size exclusion and adsorptive characteristics to retain aggregates through hydrophobic interactions. Single-use viral filtering solutions are available from a number of manufacturers, including Sartorius, Pall, and Millipore, to get rid of both tiny and big enveloped viruses. Viral elimination filters are frequently made of nano filters. These filters' most popular retention ratings are 20 or 50 nm.

4.5.4 TFF AND UF/DF FILTERS

Single-use processing works well for filtering applications. A solution's buffer can be changed and concentrated using the ultrafiltration and diafiltration processes. The active pharmaceutical ingredient is transferred to a stabilizing environment and the proper concentration is achieved during the final formulation through the use of ultrafiltration and diafiltration. Depending on whether the column eluates can be separated, processing volumes of up to 300–5,000 L would be required. Antibodies are frequently retained in membranes with a 30 kDa molecular weight threshold; the process intermediate is concentrated and diluted five times. There are modules up to $3 m^2$ in size that can process 200 L/ (h m^2). Since there are already single-use modules and pumps available, it makes sense to carry out the filtration steps in a closed system. Several single-use systems (Scilog, Millipore) are available for a limited filter area (up to 2.5 m^2). However, larger systems that might replace existing reusable systems with 14 m^2 are also possible.

Ready-to-use cassettes containing single-use TFF modules are offered for use in TFF systems. These methods offer more flexibility and speedy response. To minimize setup time, single-use systems can be purchased as preassembled units with sensors and gamma-irradiated flow pathways. A diaphragm pump with four pistons or a peristaltic pump. As a single-use part, pre-sanitized and pre-packaged cassettes are another choice. When using multiple products, cleaning a TFF system and cassette is a crucial step in the downstream process. Reducing the possibility of cross-contamination while maintaining adequate flux rates is crucial. To ensure that there is no product carryover from prior batches, cleaning procedures—even for the systems specifically designed for each product—must be thoroughly evaluated. It is possible to assemble an entirely one-time-use TFF system using readily available components (including valves, sensors, and 2D bags for liquid). Large-scale manufacturing may find it convenient to deploy automated single-use systems thanks to technological advancements and the integration of single-use components.

4.5.5 Applications for General Filtration

Reusing filters is rare in the pharmaceutical business, with the exception of steel meshes used in the mass production of nonsterile dosage forms. The first single-use parts were filter devices in biological manufacturing, mostly due to cleaning issues, even though the parts have always been reasonably priced.

The biopharmaceutical sector uses a wide range of filter types and processes. Pleated or wound filter fleeces made from melt-blown random fiber matrices are frequently used as prefilters. These filters are used to get rid of a lot of contaminants from the fluid. Prefilters can be tuned for all required applications and feature a wide range of retention ratings. Prefilters are most frequently used to safeguard membrane filters, which are more selective and tighter than prefilters. Fluids can be sterilized or polished using membrane filters. To determine whether or not these filters satisfy the performance requirements, integrity testing is required. Membranes for micro- or ultrafiltration can be used with crossflow filtration. The fluid keeps the membrane layer open by sweeping over it. The diafiltration or concentration of fluid streams is also possible with this filtration mode.

One of the simplest filter operating modes is dead-end filtration. The basic idea behind dead-end filtration is to use a pressure drop—typically created by a pump or compressed gas pressure—to move a fluid feed stream through a filter device. The filter material retains any impurities larger than the pore size of the filter media, which eventually plugs the channels or pores of the media and results in a blockage.

The setup makes little use of accessories including tanks, controllers, and tubing/piping. For sterile processing, dead-end filters with microporous membranes made of synthetic polymers such polyethersulfone, polyamide, cyanoacrylate, and polyvinylidene fluoride are widely employed. The final filtration of the purified bulk medication ingredient, bioburden reduction during cell harvest clarity, chromatography column protection, and media filtration into sterile bags and containers are all done using them. These filters are frequently pre-sterilized by gamma irradiation and arrive attached to single-use bags. By creating differential or hydrostatic pressure, pumps are utilized to move fluids; the highest pressure that may be applied depends on the bioprocess component that is least resistant to the pressure. Some unit operations, like harvesting, TFF, and chromatography, need the molecule to be very sensitive to changes in pumping. The pulsing could damage the pump's internal parts or have an impact on the fluid being pumped. The pump must have the following characteristics in order to be suitable for the use for which it is intended.

- low exposure with respect to surface area and volume
- minimum levels of leachable and extractable
- controlled flow and pressure
- minimal shear and pulsation
- absence of mechanical spalling or contact material shedding
- self-priming
- not a build-up of heat
- sterility
- increased efficacy in volume

Permanent stainless-steel process lines are complex, expensive to build, and require a lot of cleaning and validation. Because they use mechanical seals that can't maintain sterility or a consistent flow, some pumps aren't as good for handling biologics.

These days, peristaltic, syringe, and diaphragm pumps offer single-use pumping solutions. Single-use positive displacement quaternary diaphragm pumps are among the best options for bioprocessing applications. Although these volume displacement pumps are easy to use and keep the substance out of reach, they may overstress the tubing, especially if operations are prolonged. Particles generated by tension-induced erosion of the tube may contaminate the fluids being passed through. By supplying low pressure and handling biological substances gently, peristalstic pumps protect them from shear stress. However, biological products could be harmed by the quick flow through microscopic holes created by a piston pump's valve system. Even valveless piston pumps use high shear factors and pressures, which could be detrimental to biological products.

High-end peristaltic dispensing pumps now function better, thanks to improved pulsation-free pump heads, precise drive motors, and modern calibration algorithms. They are extremely accurate in terms of microliter fill volumes. Since single-use tubing is the only part in contact with the substance, it prevents cross-contamination and the need for cleaning in peristaltic pumps. Peristalstic pumps with single-use tubing offer far easier cleaning validation processes than piston pumps. On the other hand, peristaltic pumps may have problems with viscous products. The pumps lose accuracy while handling pressures higher than about 1.3 bar and are unable to handle products with viscosities more than 100 cP. Many developments in pumps intended for downstream processing, including HPLC, TFF, and VF applications (e.g., Quantum; https://www.watson-marlow.com/us-en/range/watson-marlow/single-use-pumps/quantum/), have made it possible to achieve high process yields across the pressure range. In addition to being composed of bags rather than stainless steel containers, single-use pumps frequently call for specific agitators, couplings, valves, and single-use tubing. The single-use components eliminate the need for extensive validation and reduce cleaning costs. Plug-and-play options are included with TFF applications. These pumps increase the downstream process's production by causing ultra-low shear and supplying a steady flow across the required pressure range.

A diaphragm pump is a kind of positive displacement pump that uses suitable non-return check valves in combination with the reciprocating action of a Teflon, rubber, or thermoplastic diaphragm to pump a fluid. Reciprocating connecting plates provide the power for sequential quaternary diaphragm pumps. All other liquid biologics and thick liquids are easily handled by these pumps. Some pumps can also operate with minimum shear, pulsation, and heat buildup as self-priming, dry runs, and continuous flow devices.

4.6   COMPLETE FILL-OUT OPERATIONS

Fill-finish, the last stage of the process, demands strict control over aseptic procedures without sacrificing sterility or integrity while guaranteeing effectiveness and safety. Fill-finish processes therefore usually require very advanced machinery and technology. The conventional fill-finish setup makes use of fixed systems with intricate parts that need thorough assembly, disassembly, and cleaning. For dosing and filling activities, a piston pump and a time-pressure system are frequently utilized. But in order to make sure the finished product satisfies the sterility requirements, these need to be assembled, validated CIP, and SIPed. It is more probable to guarantee that the finished product is uncompromised while lowering the risk of cross-contamination when single-use components are used for these crucial production steps. Furthermore, SUT in fill-finish can boost flexibility and shorten batch turnaround times, especially for facilities that produce different products.

Single-use solutions can be included in a conventional, fixed system. The illustration shows a fill finish setup intended for one usage, complete with installed hardware, hard-piped connections, and restricted operational flexibility (Figure 4.3).

It takes more than just putting single-use components together to successfully construct a single-use system. The success of single-use implementation and sterility assurance will depend on using providers who have expertise in validating such systems and who comprehend the need of the manufacturer's requirements to integrate and offer bespoke solutions, assure compatibility, and execute assessments. Because SUTs are simple to install, operate, and eliminate CIP/SIP, they are a flexible option for filling facilities that handle both single and multiple products. This increases facility efficiency and utilization.

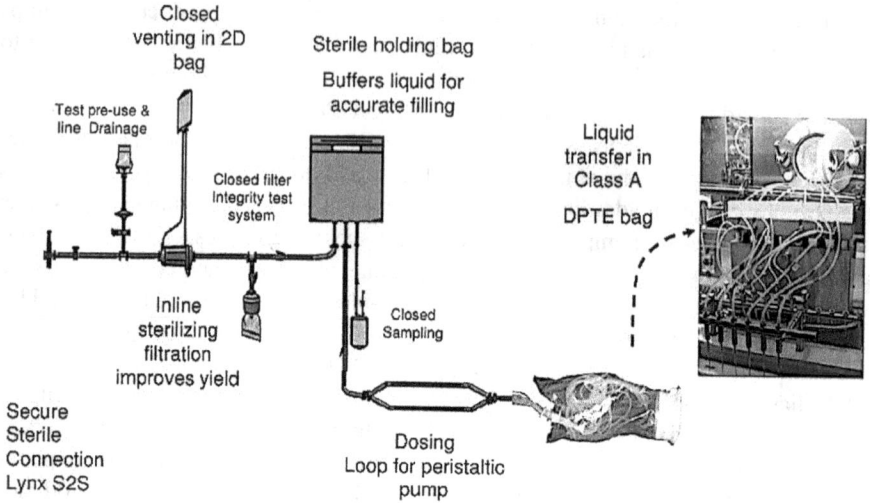

FIGURE 4.3 Closed system filling transfer set to isolator. (www.emdmillipore.com.)

4.7 SAFETY

Manufacturers of biologics are subject to regulatory requirements. This entails making certain the provider is trustworthy, able to offer the required proof of compatibility (product contact material), qualified, and validates that the single-use solutions support end-user audits. To ascertain compatibility with their process, the end-user needs to establish a user requirements specification and conduct a technical review with several vendors. Single-use parts need to be certified for the intended use in tandem with the equipment. These ought to be a part of the process validation exercise as well.

Plastic materials or elastomer systems are widely used in single-use devices, such as filter housings and the lining of bioreactors. These days, the debate regarding the potential for product contamination from chemicals in plastic film may be the biggest barrier to the broader acceptance of single-use devices. Every final container and closure must be constructed from a material that won't speed up the product's deterioration or cause it to lose its suitability for its intended purpose. (21CFR600.11 for biologics) (h)

Regulations concern the toxic effects of leachables; a risk specific to biological drugs is the impact of leachables on the three- and four-dimensional structures of protein drugs; these modifications have the potential to make the drug more immunogenic, if not less effective; as a result, the bioprocessing industry places a higher value on these side effects. Leachable chemicals are those that, throughout the manufacturing process, seep into different parts of the drug product from single-use processing equipment. In controlled research, extractables are chemical entities (both organic and inorganic) that are extracted from single-use components using standard laboratory solvents. They forecast the kinds of leachables that might be encountered during the manufacture of pharmaceuticals and reflect the worst-case scenario. It should be mentioned that leaching occurs not just with plastics but also with stainless steel, which also leaches chemicals. Stainless steel, which is frequently utilized in biopharmaceutical applications, is an alloy primarily composed of iron, nickel, and chromium with trace amounts of manganese and vanadium. It is graded 316 L. Stainless steel is a significant source of metal leaking, particularly if the surface of the tank or equipment is not adequately maintained. The elements that are most readily leachable are nickel, chromium, and iron. It has been demonstrated that when un-passivated stainless-steel vessels are stored at room temperature, much larger concentrations of metals like iron and nickel will seep into the liquid formulation than when passivated stainless steel vessels are used.

4.7.1 ADDITIVES AND POLYMERS

Single-use processing equipment for the biopharmaceutical manufacturing industry is typically made of polymers, such as plastic or rubber elastomers, as opposed to more conventional materials like metal or glass. Because polymers are lighter, more flexible, and far more durable than their conventional equivalents, they provide greater versatility. Rubber and plastic are likewise single-use materials that require no validation or cleaning. In order to add color to labels or code parts, or to clarify glass, additives can also be added to polymers. Additives are another method used to limit polymer deterioration (stabilizers).

A plastic resin's stability is affected by its molecular structure, the polymerization process, the existence of leftover catalysts, and the finishing stages employed in production. Typically, a plastic resin is treated by being put into an extruder and melted at high temperatures. Temperature, shear, and residence time in the extruder are examples of processing parameters that can have a significant impact on polymer degradation during extrusion. End-use circumstances that subject a polymer to extreme heat or light, including outdoor use or medical sterilizing procedures, might encourage polymer goods to fail too soon and lose their strength or flexibility. The end outcome, if ignored, is frequently the plastic component's complete breakdown.

In the process of making plastic, a sophisticated and challenging analysis of leachable and extractable chemical reactions takes place. These lesser-known minor chemical species may leak into a drug product when it comes to extractable and leachable testing; however, this is not always the case because it depends more on the features of the product. Polymers can leak all of their byproducts as well as additives (stabilizers, fillers, and elastomers) into pharmaceutical products.

The benefits of polymers in single-use bioprocess equipment (as well as in all medical and pharmaceutical applications) considerably exceed the hazards involved with employing additives added to polymers. Three actions will help you effectively manage these risks: choosing the right materials, putting in place an appropriate testing program, and working with vendors.

4.7.2 SELECTION OF MATERIALS

The kind of plastic that is utilized must have the necessary chemical and physical characteristics, as well as additive compatibility. Leaching can frequently be minimized by ensuring compatibility. It's crucial to choose polymers and additives that have been given the go-ahead by regulatory bodies for the intended application. As a result of the extensive analytical and toxicological testing that many substances have already undergone, a substantial quantity of information is frequently accessible about them. As a result, it is likely that most manufacturers will keep utilizing these additives, and as a result, the user does not change the composition later on because of these compounds. As major modifications in the method must be reported back to the FDA, the art of employing them is likely to endure, negating the requirement for a change control phase.

Commercially available plastic films are created using exclusive combinations and compositions; advanced scientific, for instance, uses two films to make their bags. The polyethylene film with fluid contact measures 5.0 mm. A five-layer, 7-millimeter co-extrusion film serves as the exterior layer, offering durability and protection. Table 4.3 provides an overview of the tests conducted and findings for a plastic film that is used to make bioreactor bags.

TABLE 4.3

Summary of the Tests Carried Out and Results Obtained for a Plastic Film Used to Produce Bioreactor Bags

Biocompatibility

USP Acute Systemic Injection Test	Pass	USP<88>
USP Intracutaneous Injection Test	Pass	USP<88>
USP Intramuscular Implantation Test	Pass	USP<88>
USP MEM Elution Method	Non-cytotoxic	USP<87>
Physiochemical Test for Plastics	Pass	USP <661>

Extractables

	TOC after 90 days (ppm)	pH shift after 90 days
Purified Water (pH=7)	<2	−0.79
Acidic Water (pH<2)	<3	+0.01
Basic Water (pH>10)	<4	+0.87

Physical Data

Water Vapor Transmission Rate (g/100 in²/24 hour)	0.017			ASTM F-1249
Carbon Dioxide Transmission Rate (cc/100in²/24 hour)	0.129			ASTM F-2476
Oxygen Transmission Rate (cc/100in²/24 hour)	0.023			ASTM F-1927
	Average Force	Average MOE	Average Elongation	
Tensile	32.73 lbs	25,110 psi	1,084%	ASTM D 882-02
	Min Force	Average Force	Max Force	
Tear Resistance	6.77 lbs	7.21 lbs	7.74 lbs	ASTM D1004-03
Puncture Resistance	16.42 lbs	18.61 lbs	19.51 lbs	FTMS 101C

4.8 TESTING

It is suggested that polymers used in medical and pharmaceutical applications meet USP Class VI testing requirements, as outlined in USP 88, and adhere to the relevant USP recommendations. Every bioprocessing material that comes into direct touch with the medication needs to have appropriate extractable and leachable testing processes in place.

The two-part technical guideline for assessing the risk associated with extractable and leachable materials—specifically for single-use processing equipment—provides the best-practice principles for carrying out such testing. This organization is committed to promoting the use of single-use systems and offers first-rate support and assistance. To stay up to date on the latest developments in this rapidly evolving field, readers are strongly encouraged to visit their website for updated information and take part in their numerous seminars and conventions.

When the materials have been qualified, the leachable testing process is not finished. Having a quality control program is essential as opposed to only checking the equipment or product. Risk tolerance will determine how rigorously quality control testing is conducted. Most of these leachable are probably removed during the lengthy purification processes involved in the production of recombinant pharmaceuticals. To further lower the risk, the final medium employed for protein solutions is aqueous, and many of the leachables are not soluble in water. The final packing components also represent a higher risk; for instance, rubber stoppers used to package the final dosage form have a higher probability of endangering the protein formulation than any other component to which a single-use medicine is exposed throughout the production process. Manufacturers of biologics must collaborate with suppliers to guarantee that regulatory standards are met in terms of product safety.

The DP must comply with key specifications and testing requirements, one of which is for visible and subvisible particle matter. Particulate matter contamination of medicinal products is usually effectively managed through filtration and visual inspection procedures carried out during filling. It is imperative that the single-use components are made under regulated circumstances to minimize particle matter in the final product.

4.9 REGULATORY

As it relates to extractable and leachable from single-use bioprocessing materials, there are no particular guidelines or norms. Several relevant references were written about processing materials and equipment, ignoring construction materials.

4.9.1 CANADA AND THE UNITED STATES

In Title 21 of the Code of Federal Regulations (CFR), Part 211.65, the following is introduced as the basis for the requirement to assess extractable and leachable in the United States:

Components, in-process materials, or drug products coming into touch with equipment must not be reactive, additive, or absorptive in order to change the drug product's safety, identity, strength, quality, or purity in any way that goes beyond official or other established limits.

All materials are subject to this restriction, including plastics, glass, and metals.

Although leachable may interact with a product to produce new pollutants, extractable and leachable are normally thought of as additives.

Although it was not intended for process contact materials, the US FDA's regulatory guideline for final container-closure systems provides information on the kinds of final product testing that can be done to determine what is extractable and leachable from single-use process systems and components. The FDA has determined which drug products and component dosage form interactions pose the greatest risk of extractability, and these are listed in the advice. Due in large part to the restricted amount of leachable that can be permitted in such drug delivery systems, injectable dosage forms often have the highest likelihood of the packaging component interacting with the dosage form.

Compared to oral or topical medications, pharmaceuticals intended for injection or inhalation will raise more regulatory concerns. Similar to tablets, liquid dosage forms will be subject to more stringent regulations since they dissolve more readily in liquids than in solids.

Pharmaceutical-grade materials should also fulfill or surpass industry and regulatory requirements, including those stated in USP <87> and <88>. After coming into touch with polymeric materials, mammalian cell cultures are tested for biological reactivity using USP protocols. However, because many toxicological indicators, such as subacute and chronic toxicity along with an evaluation of carcinogenic, reproductive, developmental, neurological, and immunological effects, are not evaluated, they are not regarded as sufficient regulatory documentation for extractable and leachable substances.

4.9.2 EUROPE

Rules governing the manufacturing of pharmaceutical products in the European Union contain a reference to US 21 CFR 211.65. One helpful publication on manufacturing practices is the EU, which says: "The products shouldn't be in danger from production equipment.

The components of the production apparatus that come into touch with the product must not be too reactive, additive, or absorptive, since this could compromise the product's quality and pose a risk."

A guideline addressing container-closure systems and serving as guidance for single-use process contact materials was released by the European Medicines Evaluation Agency (EMEA) at https://www.ema.europa.eu/en/documents/scientific-guideline/guideline-plastic-immediate-packaging-materials en.pdf. The information to be included about extractable and leachable comes from interaction studies, migration studies (which are similar to leachable information for those components), extraction studies (worst-case leachable), and identification of what further testing or information is needed. Next, a plan to fill in the gaps is set and put into action.

4.9.3 INTERNET SURVEILLANCE

Upstream processes like temperature, pH, pCO_2 or pO_2, and other chemical indicators are frequently monitored online. This enables continuous feeding adjustments, pH modulation, and other modifications. However, the inability to define ideal parameters for monitoring, optimize observed attributes, and modify downstream processing due to technological limitations has prevented online monitoring of the downstream process.

Nonetheless, developing online monitoring techniques to adjust the process and change the product's yield, molecular structure, and safety components has received a lot of attention in recent years. Although it is now the fastest-growing technology, its adoption is sluggish due to the legal and technological challenges associated with depending so much on data gathered online. Table 4.4 illustrates the impact of online

TABLE 4.4
The Potential Impact of Monitoring on Critical Properties, Factors, and Conditions in Downstream Processing

Critical Properties, Factors, and Conditions	Purpose/Motivation	Product Quality	Production Economy	Regulatory Compliance
Product-Related Properties				
Product activity	Immediate information on product activity during DSP	↗	↗	↗
Product variants	Evaluation and separation of different product variants	↗	↗	↗
Impurities	Assurance of sufficient removal of impurities (HCP, DNA)	↗	↗	↗
Contaminants	Detection of possible fungal, microbial, yeast bioburden	↗	↗	↗
USP media components & introduced chemicals, resin leakage	Assurance of sufficient removal of USP media components and introduced chemicals	↗	↗	↗
Economic Factors				
Investment costs of instrumentation	–	–	↘	–
Operational and maintenance costs	–	–	↘	–
Training costs of personnel	–	–	↘	–
Productivity	Productivity improvement based on monitoring	–	↗	–
Direct batch release after formulation	Batch release after final DSP step, no storage	–	↗	↗

(Continued)

TABLE 4.4 (*Continued*)

The Potential Impact of Monitoring on Critical Properties, Factors, and Conditions in Downstream Processing

Critical Properties, Factors, and Conditions	Purpose/Motivation	Product Quality	Production Economy	Regulatory Compliance
Economic Factors				
Process endpoint monitoring	Facilitation to determine the endpoint of each DSP step	↗	↗	↗
Lifetime of instrument	Usage for an extended period	–	↗	↗
Monitoring of batch-to-batch variations	Determination of batch variations and comparison to previous results (batch trajectory)	↗	↗	↗
Conditions by Regulatory Demands				
Online monitoring and process control	Possibility to fine-tune each DSP step promptly and take corrective actions	↗	↗	↗
Robustness of monitoring system	Adoption to changing process environment	↗	↗	↗
Identification of critical quality attributes	Increase process understanding and impact of CQAs in DSP steps	↗	↗	↗
Process automation	Improve process efficiency	–	↗	↗
Risk assessment	Evaluations of risks and risk-based product development	↗	↗	↗
Fulfillment of final product specifications	Ensuring quality criteria of each batch	↗	↗	↗

monitoring on downstream processing, whereas Table 4.5 presents the current state of technology. (After Patricia Roch and Carl-Fredrik Mandenius, Online monitoring of downstream bioprocesses, CURRENT OPINION IN CHEMICAL ENGINEERING, 2016, 14, pp. 112–120. http://dx.doi.org/10.1016/j.coche.2016.04.007.)

4.10 PROSPECTIVE PRODUCTION SYSTEMS

Process Intensification thus becomes a prerequisite to CM technologies that can increase tier, manage high media volumes, buffers, and generally intensify the process to extract more from the entire production process. CM is a version of highly intensified processing with brief downtimes compared to the typical time used for traditional batch production.

Because businesses can synergistically use single-use and intensification facilities that lead to reduced facility footprints and costs, the benefits of intensification and continuous processing primarily revolve around increasing productivity and reducing the need to invest in conventional, highly costly manufacturing facilities. CM is

TABLE 4.5
Technologies Used in Analytical Testing

Techniques	Biological Relevance	Sensitivity	Selectivity	Response Time	Precision	Reproducibility	Readiness for Implementation
Temperature and pressure sensors	•	•••	•	•••	•••	•••	•
pH sensor	•	•••	•	•••	•••	•••	•
Optical density	•	•	•	•••	•••	•••	•
Mass flowmeters	•	•	•	•••	•	•••	•
Dipsticks for antigens	•••	•	••	•••	•	•••	•
Flow injection analysis	••	•••	•••	••	•••	•••	•••
HPLC online	••	•••	•••	••	•••	•••	•••
Capacitive immunosensors	•••	•••	•••	•••	•••	•••	•••
Advanced mass spectrometry	•••	•••	•••	•••	•••	•••	•••
Multi fluorescence spectroscopy	••	•••	•••	•••	•••	•	
UV/VIS spectroscopy	••	•••	•••	•••	•••	•••	•••
Near-infrared spectroscopy	••	•••	•••	•••	•••	•••	•••
Mid-infrared spectroscopy	••	•••	••	•••	•••	•••	•••
Raman spectroscopy	•••	•••	•	•••	•••	•	•••
Surface Plasmon Resonance	•••	•••	•••	•	(•)	••	•••
Capillary electrophoresis online	••	•••	•••	••	•••	••	
Flow cytometry online	••	•••	•••	•	•••	•••	•••
NMR online	•••	•••	•••	••	•••	•••	•••
Offline biosensors	•••	•••	•••	••	•••	•••	••
Circular Dichroism	•••	•••	••	••	•••	•••	•••
Light scattering	••	•••	•	••	•••	•••	•••

Source: After Roch, P.; Mandenius, C.-F. Online monitoring of downstream bioprocesses, *Curr. Opin. Chem. Eng.*, 2016, 14, 112–120. https://doi.org/10.1016/j.coche.2016.04.007.

a crucial step in promoting drug quality and enhancing production efficiency, which in turn results in lower drug prices.

The idea of connected manufacturing, in which unit operations are physically and, most significantly, even digitally integrated, is one of the main forces behind the effective integration of CM (automated). Employing a completely connected and integrated system that can regulate and track product quality helps to expedite the process from beginning to end.

Enhancing product quality has the advantage of saving time for certain unit operations that might otherwise result in deterioration or additional variations. Examples of these operations include the bioreactor process and chromatography separation, which can successfully resolve the product's other variants (isoforms). A perfusion bioreactor connected to a multi-column chromatography capture step, flow-through virus inactivation, multi-column intermediate purification, a flow-through membrane adsorber polishing step, continuous VF, and a final ultrafiltration step run in continuous mode are a few examples of continuous biomanufacturing processes. The widespread use of continuous capture steps is mostly attributable to the advancements in multi-column chromatography, which are perfect for large-scale production.

One step toward cutting waste and simplifying processes for increased efficiency is the implementation of CM operations. Even though the idea may be relatively new or, more accurately, underutilized in the field of biological medicine, it is still necessary to adapt other downstream processes, including UF/DF. Although this is a difficulty, one approach is to use sterile UF capsules, which provides the simple installation and operation of closed systems with little concerns of contamination or bioburden. To further design UF/DF operations to a continuous approach, automation for process monitoring and data collecting in conjunction with single-use technology is taken into consideration. Single-pass TFF systems are becoming more and more popular, and they are useful single-use options. Nevertheless, there is clearly a great deal of room for improvement with these commercial-scale skids and recipes that call for high product concentration.

Recognizing the requirement for continuous processing and outlining the specifics of how the batch process might be modified or converted into a continuous one are the first steps in implementing the concept. Since not all batch operations are intended to be continuous, it might not be simple to convert a batch operation from the start to a continuous operation. Batch processing is a multi-step process that is supported by both online and offline analyses that establish the control approach. Therefore, it could be simpler to convert just a few phases at first, but modifications should only be made if they preserve or boost productivity and have no detrimental effects on the quality of the final output.

A more sensible and sensible step toward implementing CM is to use a hybrid approach to continuous biomanufacturing, in which only the upstream or a portion of the downstream process is run continuously. This can be done by running a fed-batch process with a continuous chromatography capture step or by running upstream as a perfusion operation coupled with batch mode purification.

The regulators are also becoming more supportive of continuous production. The FDA's proposal for continuous unit operations is evidence that the processing of biological medicines is moving in the direction of a future that supports developing technology. Reducing product failure, raising quality, and boosting efficiency are the driving forces behind the demand. This serves to support ongoing initiatives aimed at automation, stepping up procedures, and efficiently using resources (facility and equipment).

4.10.1 CONTINUOUS CHROMATOGRAPHY OPERATIONS

Systems for continuous chromatography are made for processing in real time, mainly when the purification step is connected to an upstream bioreactor perfusion or simply a basic fed-batch procedure. When using batch chromatography, each purification step is carried out using a single, sizable column. A continuous multi-column setup efficiently manages operations across several smaller columns simultaneously by operating them in series over several cycles. One or more columns may be in the wash, elution, or regeneration stages while the other(s) is/are being loaded with product. An alternative is to divide the loading stage between two series-connected columns.

With the assistance and encouragement of regulators, continuous chromatography is attracting a lot of attention in moving the process toward clinical development and is more likely to be produced on a commercial scale. By utilizing small-to-medium-sized columns, inline dilution capabilities, lower buffer usage, and bioreactors that can support high productivity, continuous chromatography operations can assist reduce the footprint of their facilities. Protein A resin capacity can be better utilized and these potential benefits can be realized with the aid of multi-column chromatography. A continuous chromatographic capture stage can be integrated with a fed-batch process to save expenses and time while potentially increasing product quality. There are still issues to be resolved, nevertheless, because of the increased sophistication of hardware systems and certain alleged regulatory complications.

However, each project is given a thorough evaluation based on the operational scale, characteristics, and other process requirements of the protein before determining whether continuous chromatography is the best option. It might not always be feasible to quickly implement a continuous end-to-end system, and it's not always simple to transition from batch to continuous processing. However, newer technologies that can be employed as continuous or semi-continuous processing options in place of traditional batch processing include straight-through processing (STP), simulated moving bed (SMB), and PCC.

4.10.2 PROCESSING DIRECTLY THROUGH STP

STP involves connecting two or more chromatographic processes in series and adjusting process conditions in line between columns to guarantee ideal loading conditions for the subsequent step. This arrangement would eliminate the need for intermediary

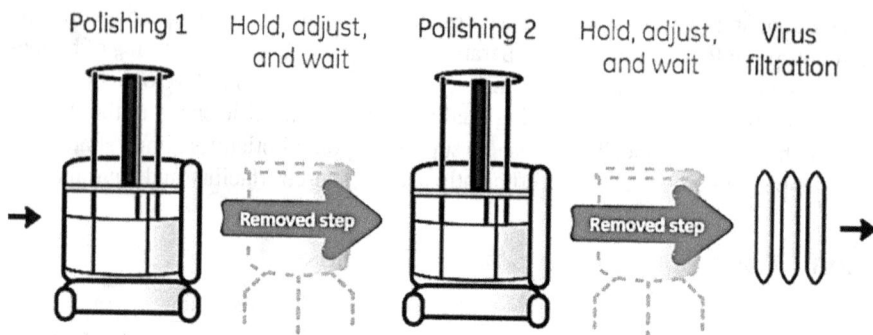

FIGURE 4.4   By connecting the filter and purification systems in series and moving adjustments in line, the overall equipment footprint can be decreased. (Cytiva Life Sciences.)

conditioning stages that are necessary for batch operations that are typical, meaning that little to no intermediate hold-up tanks would be needed, increasing efficiency and requiring less equipment (Figure 4.4).

4.10.3   PERIODIC CHROMATOGRAPHY WITH COUNTERCURRENTS (PCC)

PCC is a multi-step method that reduces resin volume and maximizes the utilization of chromatography resin capacity while decreasing process time. PCC leverages the resin capacity by completing three or more column chromatography procedures. After loading Column 1 to a 60%–80% breakthrough, it is disconnected in order to carry out the equilibration, wash, and elution procedures. Meanwhile, Column 2 is brought up to breakthrough and the process is shifted to it. Next come the steps of disconnecting, washing, eluting, and equilibrating, and finally repeating the process with Column 3. Column 1 is now prepared to resume these operations online, enabling continuous processing. This makes it possible to use more of the available resin while requiring less equipment and enabling efficient time management.

4.10.4   SMB CHROMATOGRAPHY

Applications for SMB chromatography include the food and petrochemical sectors. It is distinguished by enabling processes to attain high productivity in comparison to batch methods because of the effective use of the liquid and solid phases needed for separation.

The fundamental idea of simulated moving bed chromatography is to create a countercurrent flow by moving the solid adsorbent (beds) in several smaller columns that hold them in the opposite direction of the fluid (feed, eluent, and product). Multiport valves positioned in between the columns are usually used to provide the "simulated movement," allowing the feed, eluent, and product fluid streams to be periodically transferred from column to column in the direction of fluid flow. The placement and control of the valves aid in the strategic movement of the sample and solvent, enabling many columns to execute separate stages of separation concurrently as a continuous cycle.

4.10.5 CONTINUOUS MANUFACTURING

The industrial standard for recombinant protein technology is the batch method, or CM. But if the protein is secreted into a growth medium, it can also be generated in a vessel from which the yield is continually extracted. Importantly, it keeps cells at greater viabilities and helps to increase the output of labile proteins by preventing inconsistent post-translational modifications. Significant savings are also added by the decreased testing in addition to the material expenses (Figure 4.5).

Although there has been a long-standing effort to develop a CM process, the FDA didn't publish its first guidance on the subject until March 2023. This guidance addressed the legal and scientific concerns that come up during the development, implementation, and management of CM for chemical and biological drugs. A therapeutic protein's production pathway in a CM is depicted in Figure 4.2. The FDA lists other regulations that govern CM.

The CM system for therapeutic proteins is shown in Figure 4.5 (FDA Source).

A bioreactor that is compatible with a perfusion culture system, continuous capture chromatography, VF, virus inactivation, buffer exchange, and buffer concentration using tangential flow chromatography columns are some of the unit activities that make up the setup. Every unit operation is connected to other unit operations via

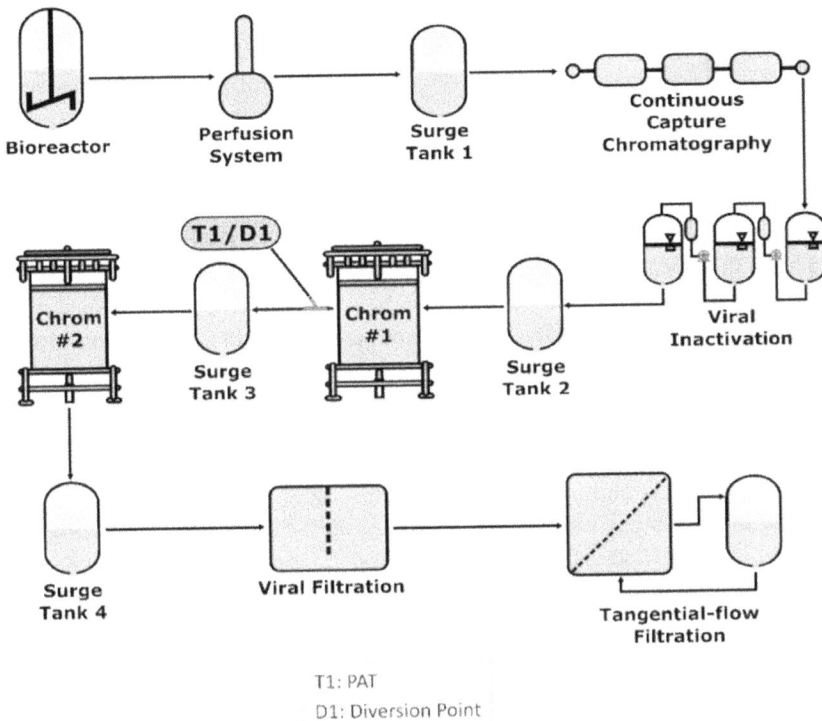

T1: PAT
D1: Diversion Point

FIGURE 4.5   Continuous manufacturing system for therapeutic proteins. (FDA.)

a surge line, tank, or adjacent unit operation integration. Following chromatography, PAT (T1) and diversion sites D1 are found (Chrom #1). Continuous operations can be made to account for variations in mass flow rates or process dynamics by using a surge line or tank. When needed, the unit operations can be combined.

CM, independent of material type, is the continuous feeding of input materials into, transformation of materials in-process within, and simultaneous removal of materials output from a manufacturing process in an integrated system with two or more unit operations. The amount of input material, the amount of output material, and the run time (minimum or maximum) at a specified mass flow rate are the parameters that determine the batch size generated by CM. A single thaw of one or more vials from the same cell bank in CM procedures can yield one or more harvests. It should be mentioned how many or what range of cell bank vials are used to make the designated medicinal substance batches. The output drug substance batches should be linked to the cell bank vials. Biosimilar developers may now appropriately plan the process shift because the FDA advice outlines how the eCTD file should be managed for the CM procedure. Proteins that are secreted or engineered to secrete in *E. Coli* can be treated using this method (Table 4.6).

The goal of maximizing manufacturing costs through CM of chemical and biological products has long been in place; however, cGMP compliance issues delayed its implementation until March 2023, when the FDA released its first guideline on the development and application of CM, especially for biological products. A perfusion system is needed for CM, and *E. Coli* is a better option than CHO cells because its batch cycle is typically considerably shorter—a few hours as opposed to weeks—instead of weeks for CHO cells. There are multiple options for rerouting the recombinant protein in *E. coli*, utilizing the characteristics of each cellular compartment and the protein produced. The proteins can be guided to the cytoplasm, periplasm, or released directly into culture media.

For a number of years, efforts have been made to find a CM method.

The FDA expects a lot of interest even though it hasn't yet approved a biological product made in a continuous system. The FDA consequently published its first advice on CM in March 2023, addressing the scientific and regulatory concerns that surfaced during the development, implementation, running, and lifecycle management of CM for chemical and biological pharmaceuticals, including the eCTD filing structure. This guideline has made it possible to switch from batch systems to continuous systems, which will have a substantial impact on the cost of development and manufacturing, the stability of proteins, and the size of the bioreactors.

A therapeutic protein's production pathway in a CM is depicted in Figure 4.5. The FDA lists other regulations that govern CM. The industrial standard for recombinant protein technology is the batch procedure. But if the protein is secreted into the growth medium, it can also be generated in a vessel from which the yield is continually extracted. Importantly, it keeps cells at greater viabilities and helps to increase the output of labile proteins by preventing inconsistent PTMs. Significant savings are also added by the decreased testing in addition to the material expenses.

While CM is mostly intended for mammalian cells, *E. coli* also secretes proteins (Table 4.6), allowing using of both prokaryote and eukaryote systems suitable for CM.

TABLE 4.6
Therapeutic Proteins that *E. Coli* Secretes

Adiponectin receptor
Adiponectin
Alpha-amylase
Amylase
Antibacterial peptides
Antibodies
Antithrombin III
Bone morphogenetic protein (BMP)
Chimeric antigen receptor (CAR)
Cholecystokinin (CCK)
Chymosin (rennin)
Ciliary neurotrophic factor (CNTF)
Coagulation factor VIII
Colony-stimulating factor 1 (CSF-1)
Connective tissue growth factor (CTGF)
Epidermal growth factor (EGF)
Erythropoietin (EPO)
Erythropoietin receptor (EPOR)
Factor IX
Factor VII
Factor VIII
Fibrinolytic enzymes
Fibroblast growth factor (FGF)
Follicle-stimulating hormone (FSH)
Glucagon-like peptide-1 (GLP-1)
Glucagon
Glucocerebrosidase
Glucokinase
Glutathione S-transferase (GST)
Granulocyte colony-stimulating factor (G-CSF)
Granulocyte colony-stimulating factor receptor (G-CSF receptor)
Granulocyte-macrophage colony-stimulating factor (GM-CSF)
Green fluorescent protein (GFP)
Growth hormone (GH)
Hepatitis B surface antigen (HBsAg)
Hepatitis B surface antigen (HBsAg)
Human calcitonin
Human growth factor-1 (HGF-1)
Human growth hormone receptor antagonist (GHR antagonist)
Insulin-like growth factor 1 (IGF-1)
Insulin-like growth factor 2 (IGF-2)
Insulin-like growth factor-binding protein (IGFBP)
Insulin

(Continued)

TABLE 4.6 *(Continued)*
Therapeutic Proteins that *E. Coli* Secretes

Interferon alpha-2b
Interferon beta-1a
Interferon gamma (IFN-γ)
Interferon-alpha (IFN-α)
Interferon-beta (IFN-β)
Interferon-gamma (IFN-γ)
Interferon-lambda (IFN-λ)
Interleukin-1 receptor antagonist (IL-1RA)
Interleukin-10 (IL-10)
Interleukin-11 (IL-11)
Interleukin-12 (IL-12)
Interleukin-13 (IL-13)
Interleukin-15 (IL-15)
Interleukin-17 (IL-17)
Interleukin-18 (IL-18)
Interleukin-2 (IL-2)
Interleukin-2 (IL-2)
Interleukin-4 (IL-4)
Interleukin-5 (IL-5)
Interleukin-6 (IL-6)
Lactoferrin
Leptin
Lipase
Matrix metalloproteinases (MMPs)
Nerve growth factor (NGF)
Nerve growth factor beta (NGF-β)
Nerve growth factor receptor (NGF receptor)
Oncolytic viruses
Osteopontin
Parathyroid hormone (PTH)
Platelet-derived growth factor (PDGF)
Relaxin-2
Relaxin
Serine protease
Somatostatin receptor
Streptavidin
Streptococcal M protein
Streptokinase
Thrombopoietin (TPO)
Tissue plasminogen activator (tPA)
Transforming growth factor-beta (TGF-β)
Vascular endothelial growth factor (VEGF)

5 Strategic Understanding for Biosimilars Future

5.1 INTRODUCTION

The time-to-entry of biosimilar development is 5–9 years, and the average cost reaches $100–$300 million [1–4]. The reason for the wide range comes from the differences in types of products. For example, cytokines such as erythropoietin and Granulocyte colony stimulating factor (GCSF) require much less time and lower costs than the mAbs used to treat cancer.

Thus far, the FDA has approved 44 biosimilars composed of only 12 molecules (tocilizumab, bevacizumab, etanercept, epoetin alfa, trastuzumab, adalimumab, insulin glargine, ranibizumab, pegfilgrastim, filgrastim, infliximab, rituximab, ustekinumab, and natalizumab). At the same time, more than 200 licensed proteins [5], almost half of them with expired patents [6], await entry.

Figure 5.1 shows the broad distribution of the cost of development of biosimilars. The discussion below investigates the five cost categories and offers solutions that can reduce the overall price by 90% and the time by at least 50%. These are not suggestions for shortcuts that might compromise safety and efficacy; these are suggestions based on scientific and rational facts that are currently well-proven.

Biosimilars are to biological drugs, what the generics are to chemical drugs. When the laws were enacted for chemical drugs, such as the Hatch-Waxman Act: The Drug Price Competition and Patent Term Restoration Act of 1984, the drugs manufactured by a biological entity, such as an animal cell line, were excluded since it is not possible to ensure an identical chemical structure and, therefore, it is not possible to ascertain their equivalence based on chemistry alone [8]. It took 25 years to create another law in the US to address the generic forms of biological drugs labeled as biosimilars to avoid any confusion with chemical drugs. But legislative vested interests marred this effort, and it required the FDA to reclassify therapeutic proteins and bring them to the Center for Drug Evaluation and Research (CDER) from the Center for Biologics Evaluation and Research (CBER) that dealt with drugs or other products manufactured by a biological entity [9]. The approval process, however, kept its label as "licensing," as more rigorous testing, and at one time, it had required a license to manufacture antibiotics. A biologics license application (BLA) is a request for permission to introduce or deliver, for introduction, a biologic product into interstate commerce (21 CFR 601.2). The BLA is regulated under 21 CFR 600–680.

After several years of legislative attempts, the Biologics Price Control and Innovations Act (BPCIA) of 2019 [10] was finally approved in 2010 [11] as SEC 7001 [12] of the Patient Protection and Affordable Care Act (BPCIA) [13]. Under the BPCIA, "biological product" refers to proteins, except chemically produced polypeptides. Biological goods are recombinant proteins that are naturally generated and

DOI: 10.1201/9781003404637-5

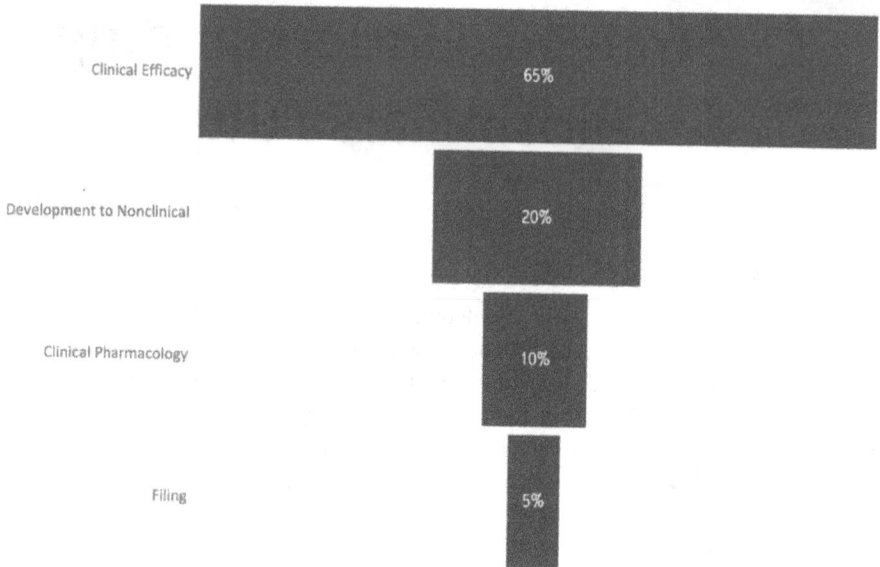

FIGURE 5.1 Cost distribution of testing of 246 biosimilars approved in the US, EU, and Japan from 2006 to 2021 [7]. The filing cost also includes the "patent dance" cost in the US.

have approved NDAs. Furthermore, a biosimilar that is the focus of "an application submitted under subsection (k)" may use only a "single biological product licensed under subsection (a)" as a reference product. Otherwise, neither an FD&CA protein nor a biosimilar may be used as a reference product in a 351(k) application. When H.R.3590—The Patient Protection and Affordable Care Act was introduced on 09/17/2009 [12], it did not mention biosimilars until it was ordered to be printed on 11/19/2009; it then included the term "biosimilar" 36 times and included all clauses of the previous bills. It is important to understand the history of legislative actions that have led to the current BPCIA to identify what amendments should be made further to bring more biosimilars to patients.

Differing from section 505g of the FD&CA [14], Representative Waxman's first biosimilars bill, RR 6257 [15], was more akin to section 505(b)(2) and allowed a case-by-case approach regarding clinical and other data supporting licensure of biosimilars. The bill was introduced in September 2006 in the House. The law offered an alternative strategy for patent litigation and would not have granted data exclusivity for novel products. It was highly significant that two approaches were proposed to approve biosimilars.

The Public Health Safety Act (PHSA) [16] permits the FDA to license "comparable" biological products, as per section 351(k)(l). The criteria for approving modifications to the chemistry, production, or quality assurance of authorized pharmaceuticals and biological products are called "comparable."

Second, the agency was permitted to license biological products "[differing] from or incorporating a change to a licensed reference product" under section 351(k)(2), even if the products were not comparable, provided that the safety, purity, and potency of the proposed product were demonstrated "relative to the reference product." It appears that the FDA's interpretation of section 505(b)(2) of the FD&CA served as the model for section 351(k)(2). However, this clause was removed from the BPCIA.

To obtain licensure under the proposed section 351(k)(l), an applicant would have needed to show that the reference product and its proposed product were "comparable." The evidence of this was based on (i) data from biological, chemical, and physical assays and "other non-clinical laboratory studies" and (ii) data generated in "any necessary clinical study or studies sufficient to confirm safety, purity, and potency in one or more appropriate conditions of use." Any required clinical studies were "designed to avoid duplicative and unethical clinical testing." The FDA could not require post-marketing studies as a condition of approval.

The BPCIA does not mention "necessary" and "duplicative and unethical" clinical testing. Adding these terms back in would reawaken the argument that if efficacy testing cannot fail, it is unnecessary and thus unethical [17].

HR 6257 would have directed the FDA to find various products, including proteins with minor differences in their amino acid sequence, to have "comparable principle molecular structural features." Examples were drawn from a similar list in FDA regulations implemented following the Orphan Drug Act. The list was as follows: (i) two proteins with structural differences "solely due to post-translational events, infidelity of translation or transcription, minor differences in amino acid sequence"; (ii) two polysaccharides with similar saccharide repeating units, even if there were differences in the number of units and polymerization modifications; (iii) two glycosylated proteins, if the differences between them was solely due to posttranslational events, the infidelity of transcription or translation, or "minor differences in amino acid sequence" and, in cases where the proteins had similar saccharide repeating units, even if there were differences in the number of units and postpolymerization modifications; (iv) two polynucleotide products having an identical sequence of purine and pyrimidine bases or their derivatives and an identical sugar backbone; and (v) "closely related, complex partly definable drugs with similar therapeutic intent, such as two live viral products for the same indication." This extensive description was removed even though it would have been the foundation of later suggestions requiring the FDA to create monographs of biological drugs.

Like the current BPCIA, HR 6257 would have created a scheme for identifying and resolving patent issues related to the market entry of comparable biological products.

Waxman's second bill, HR 1038 [18], was introduced during the 110th Congress. It was different from his first bill in several respects. On April 19, 2007, Representative Jay Inslee introduced the "Patient Protection and Innovative Biologic Medicines Act of 2007" [19]. Just over a month later, Senator Judd Gregg introduced a similar bill, the "Affordable Biologics for Consumers Act," S. 1505 [20]. However, the two bills bore a "strong resemblance" and shared elements with the EU model. Like the second Waxman bill, HR 1038, HR 1956, and S. 1505 would have added subsection (k) to the Public Health Service Act (PHSA) section 351 to create a pathway for the licensure of biosimilars.

Under both the Gregg bill and the Inslee bill, the new pathway would have been available for biosimilars under section 351(a) or approved based on an application submitted under FD&CA section 505(b)(l). This approach was broader than the approach in the first two Waxman bills because it permitted FD&CA-approved proteins to serve as reference products. Biosimilar versions of these proteins would have been subject to the new pathway rather than sections 505g or 505(b)(2). The Waxman bill permitted only products with an approved BLA to serve as reference products and would have left open section 505(b)(2) and (theoretically) section 505g for the approval of biosimilar versions of FD&CA proteins. The approaches of the Inslee and Gregg bills were narrower than that of the second Waxman bill insofar as they applied only to therapeutic proteins, not other PHSA biologics, such as vaccines and blood products; the former bills' approaches were also similar in some respects to the EU approach [21].

Under the Waxman bill, the FDA would have determined the necessary data for the licensure of a comparable biological product on a case-by-case basis through private negotiations with the applicant. Under both bills, the data requirements for a given "product class" of biosimilars would have been established through a public process. In the case of HR 1956, this process was guidance development, and in the case of S. 1505, it was rulemaking. Both bills described minimum data requirements for biosimilar applications. The Inslee bill would have established a procedure for adopting product class-specific guidance. It also would have mandated that all product class-specific guidance documents call for the inclusion of a postmarketing safety monitoring plan. In contrast, the Gregg bill would have required information about the "post-market assessment and monitoring" of the biosimilar's safety, purity, and potency.

Under HR 1956 [19], the FDA could have approved a section 351(k) application if the applicant showed that a similar biological product met the applicable product class-specific guidance requirements. Neither bill would have permitted submission of a section 351(k) application until the FDA published the final product class-specific guidance or rule and 12 years had elapsed since the licensure of the reference product.

In contrast to the Hatch-Waxman bill and HR 1038 [18], the Inslee bill contained no patent provisions. The Inslee bill took an approach like that employed in Europe, where patent infringement issues must be litigated after generic and biosimilar market entry.

Under the Gregg bill [20], the FDA could have approved a biosimilar application once the data exclusivity period expired, regardless of whether patent litigation had concluded. Nevertheless, if a patent was found valid and infringed upon before biosimilar licensure (presumably by any court, although this was not explicitly stated), the FDA could not have approved [20] the application until the patent's expiry. The bill also provided that the biosimilar applicant could not initiate a declaratory judgment regarding a patent identified by the patent owner in its initial notice after (i) the date 18 months before the expiration of the data exclusivity period or (ii) the date 60 days after the provision of the written explanation if that occurred during the last 18 months before data exclusivity expired.

The S. 1695 [11] added, "notwithstanding minor differences in clinically inactive components." Additionally, the bill called for data from animal studies, although the phrasing was later modified to include "animal toxicology," which was replaced with "nonclinical testing" in 2022. The language "to avoid needlessly duplicative or unethical clinical testing" was later removed from the BPCIA.

The interchangeability criteria included in S. 1956 departed from every prior approach in that a single-use product would meet the standard for interchangeability if it could "be expected to produce the same clinical result as the reference product in any given patient." For products intended to be used more than once, the applicant would have also been required to demonstrate that the risk to patients regarding the safety or diminished efficacy from switching between the two products was no greater than the risk from the exclusive use of the reference product.

This chapter presents a brief history of biosimilar development and legislation, along with specific suggestions for the actions that the US Congress, the FDA, and developers could take that should lead to time and cost savings of more than 80% to secure approval of biosimilars, the only way, the products can become affordable, to meet the intention of the BPCIA.

5.2   THE ROLE OF THE US CONGRESS

The first amendment to the BPCIA was made toward the end of 2022, with the term "animal toxicology" in Section (bb) being removed and replaced with "nonclinical testing" as part of The FDA Modernization Act [22,23], which further clarified that the amendment:

> Authorizes the use of certain alternatives to animal testing, including cell-based assays and computer models, to obtain an exemption from the Food and Drug Administration to investigate the safety and effectiveness of a drug. It also removes a requirement to use animal studies as a part of the process to obtain a license for a biological product that is biosimilar or interchangeable with another biological product.

This amendment's scientific foundation was the realization that animals might not have the receptors needed for biological medications to function. Nevertheless, a description of this uncertainty remained lacking in the FDA Modernization Act 2.0, as stated by the Medicines and Healthcare Products Regulatory Agency (MHRA) [24]:

> No in vivo animal studies are requested as these are not relevant for showing comparability between a biosimilar candidate and its RP: this includes pharmacodynamic, kinetic, and toxicity studies.[24]

One impact of this amendment that may not be fully understood is that animal studies cannot be used to justify any differences in the analytical profile of a biosimilar product, such as the presence of unmatched impurities, as had been done in the past.

5.2.1   INTERCHANGEABILITY

The US is one of the few countries, including Brazil, Cuba, Ghana, Peru, Russia, and Zambia, requiring extensive clinical testing to allow interchangeability. Most other countries leave this to the prescriber's discretion or allow automatic substitution [25,26]. To secure interchangeable status, switching studies are designed to include at least three switches, with two alternating exposures to the candidate drug. Across the arms of a switching study, the primary endpoints typically evaluate the pharmacodynamics of the compound. In contrast, the secondary endpoints are safety, efficacy, and immunogenicity (the generation of anti-drug antibodies).

Since interchangeability is a legislative requirement, this status can only be removed by amending the BPCIA. However, the FDA can play a pivotal role in exploiting the exclusivity provision to encourage the admission of many new biosimilars; this can be accomplished by the FDA awarding interchangeability to all products but giving the first product a 12-month exclusivity period before another biosimilar can be given this classification. This will bring a deluge of filings of biosimilars.

5.2.2 PATENT LITIGATION

The FDA is required by the Hatch-Waxman Act to receive a list of patents from small-molecule reference drug manufacturers that indicates the compositions, formulations, active ingredients, and treatment methods of their approved reference drug products (DPs). The FDA must then publish this list in its "Orange Book" Section 355(b)(1), (c) of 21 USC (2). All applicants for generic drugs are thus provided with advance notice of the patents that may be asserted by a reference drug producer in future Hatch-Waxman litigation by the patents' inclusion in the FDA Orange Book.

However, until recently, reference product sponsors (RPSs) were not required under the BPCIA to link the patents publicly to their licensed biologic products. The BPCIA's rules at 42 USC 262(l) controlling the prelitigation information exchanges between a specific RPS and a specific biosimilar applicant (together known as the "patent dance") were broadly consistent with the absence of such public patent disclosure requirements in the BPCIA. Under those regulations, the FDA is not involved in these voluntary, nonpublic exchanges, which include the RPS's patents and manufacturing details regarding the biosimilar applicant's product. Therefore, biosimilar manufacturers not currently engaged in a patent dance with an RPS cannot predict which patents the RPS may bring up in upcoming BPCIA litigation.

The patent dance remains one of the biggest financial and administrative obstacles to biosimilar approval. Out of 234 proposed bills, the US Congress has passed [27] 25 directly regarding biosimilars; 100 of these bills deal with the patents used to approve biosimilars, and 18 have become laws [28].

The difference between the BPCIA and Hatch-Waxman regimes has now somewhat narrowed. The Biological Product Patent Transparency (BPPT) modifications to the BPCIA became effective on June 25, 2021. The Consolidated Appropriations Act, HR 133, Pub. L. No. 116–260 included the BPPT amendments, which mandate that the FDA publish specific data regarding biologic products. The most important of these data is a list of all the patents that the RPS owns or has exclusive licensing rights to and that the RPS has previously designated as being a part of the patent dance under 42 USC 262(l)(3)(A) or (l)(7). The revelation of these hitherto undisclosed patent data carries strategic ramifications for biosimilars and RPS applicants.

The length of the exclusivity periods for interchangeable and unexpired reference products must be specified in the Purple Book. Importantly, the act mandates that the designated exclusivity periods cover only the 12-year exclusivity period for reference goods and that the exclusivity provided to biosimilar products can be interchanged.

The cost of litigation related to patents for generic drugs is approximately $3–5 million depending on the following: the features of the DP, the drug substance (DS), the method of use, and whether the case concerns a challenge to the patent's validity, patent infringement, or both [29]. For biosimilars, the costs are higher due to the complexity of the products [30]. Over 38 lawsuits have been filed for almost every biosimilar product, and most have been resolved, except for the four most recent filings [6].

While the Supreme Court has concluded that a patent dance is not required, its continued impact on litigation remains a significant issue. (20)

15–1039, 15–1195, the Supreme Court held that the patent dance is not mandatory. Although the BPCIA requires that an applicant 'must' provide its application and manufacturing information, the statute also "provides a remedy for an applicant's failure to turn over its application and manufacturing information".

Ideally, the patent dance should be amended to limit infringement claims to patents reported in the Purple Book but independently of the certificate by the biosimilar developer. This will require creating a hybrid of Paragraph IV requirements. The reason for this recommendation comes from the diversity of patents that can be involved, from gene design to upstream, downstream, formulation, and delivery systems.

5.2.3 Reference Product

A biosimilar is allowed only the approved indications of the reference product. However, over time, many possibilities have arisen to add new indications, new dosing, and even new routes of administration, all of which are not allowed in the BPCIA. These changes to the utility of an approved biosimilar require refiling the drug as a new biological drug under 351(a), adding to the cost of hundreds of millions of dollars. Since the target molecules have already had their safety established in the reference product or a biosimilar product, a new classification of filing as proposed in previous versions of BPCIA, 351(k)(2) should be revived [31]. Doing so is crucial since biological drugs have multiple modes of action that can be discovered using newer discovery methods, such as AI-based drug discovery [32]. The more recent applications can significantly change healthcare if allowed without treating the submission as a new drug for safety evaluation.

These amendments to the BPCIA should allow applicants to cite, as reference products, both innovative products and products licensed under the new pathway. This is because it defined "reference product" to include biological products licensed under section 351(a) of the (innovative biological products) and those licensed under section 351(k) (biosimilars). This early wisdom of the Waxman bill should be revisited based on the rationality of the transitive law [33]; if a biosimilar is licensed similarly to a 351(a) biological product, the biosimilar could serve as a reference product. This argument was presented in opposition to maintaining the monopoly of the RPSs.

To understand the rationality of the suggestions made above, we need to examine the transitive law, also known as the transitive property law, which is a fundamental concept in mathematics and logic asserting that if a relation holds between a first and a second element and between the second and a third element, then it necessarily has between the first and the third element as well [34]. The philosophical foundations of this concept can be traced back to the works of Aristotle and, later, Gottfried Wilhelm Leibniz. Aristotle, predating the Stoics, was interested in conditional claims and their implications [35]. The transitive law states that if A is related to B and B is related to C, then A is related to C. Thus, a biosimilar can be allowed as a reference product, and this classification would remove many constraints in securing the supply of the reference product.

5.2.4 New Biosimilars

The biosimilar approach can also apply to products other than therapeutic proteins. Still, the FDA is silent on this possibility, while the European Medicines Agency (EMA) has taken steps to allow biosimilar mRNA and gene therapy products [21]. Such differences between the US and the rest of the agencies come from the strict legislative requirement to make any change in the US, as did the BPCIA, a law that presents many inconsistencies and scientific challenges. One such element is the exclusivity of 12 years for a new product approved under 351(a) of the legislation; in the EU and UK, these limits are 8–10 years [36], but this is not the major issue that remains the high cost and time to develop biosimilars requiring testing that can be redundant.

5.2.5 Pharmacy Benefits Managers (PBMs)

Pharmacy Benefit Managers (PBMs) play a complex role in the healthcare system, and their influence on drug pricing can be a contentious issue. Here are some ways PBMs can push the cost of drugs higher [37]:

Rebates and Negotiations: PBMs negotiate drug prices for health insurance plans with pharmaceutical manufacturers. While they may secure discounts and rebates, these negotiations are often opaque and can lead to higher drug list prices. Manufacturers may increase their list prices to offset the negotiated discounts and rebates.

Formulary Placement: PBMs create formularies and lists of preferred drugs for insurance plans. Pharmaceutical companies may pay PBMs to place their drugs on these formularies, effectively giving them preferential treatment. This can limit competition and lead to higher prices for non-preferred drugs.

Spread Pricing: PBMs often charge insurance plans more for a drug than they reimburse pharmacies for dispensing it. The difference, known as the spread, can lead to higher costs for insurance plans and patients.

Generic Suppression: PBMs may favor brand-name drugs over generic alternatives, which can be more expensive. This can discourage lower-cost generics and contribute to higher drug costs.

Pharmacy Steering: PBMs may direct patients to use specific pharmacies they have contracts with, known as preferred pharmacies. This can limit patients' choices and potentially lead to higher costs if the selected pharmacy charges more for the drug.

Lack of Transparency: The lack of transparency in PBM practices makes it difficult for stakeholders, including patients and providers, to understand how drug prices are determined entirely. This lack of transparency can contribute to higher drug costs.

The complexity of their operations and potential conflicts of interest have raised concerns about their role in driving up drug prices in the United States. Efforts to increase transparency and regulate PBM practices aim to address some of these issues and reduce the overall cost of prescription drugs. The US Congress has entered over 148 bills that would require controlling the role of PBMs [38], and only one bill [39] has reached the negotiation stage, thus only remotely affecting PBMs. This indicates the strength of the PBM lobby. Even though PBMs are not listed as a critical issue for generic products, the stakes are much higher for biological drugs; the impact of PBMs must be diluted if the cost difference between biosimilars and patients is to be substantially reduced.

5.3 THE ROLE OF THE FDA

Like any other regulatory agency, the FDA has no reason to deviate from the path defined in legislation. Aside from the legislative changes suggested above, the FDA can alter the interpretation of the BPCIA to significantly increase biosimilars' entry into the US.

While the FDA has the authority to interpret the BPCIA:

DETERMINATION BY SECRETARY. —The Secretary may determine, in the Secretary's discretion, that an element described in clause (i)(I) is unnecessary in an application submitted under this subsection.

While the BPCIA requires that a biosimilar be shown to be similar to its locally licensed originator (that is, a product approved under Sect. 351(a) of the Public Health Service Act of 1942, as amended), it also expressly gives the FDA discretion to vary the information required to establish biosimilarity [See 42 USC 262(k)(2)(A)(ii)].

However, this authority does not extend to clauses of the BPCIA such as patent litigation, interchangeability, and the introduction of repurposed biologicals in a separate category, although concessions were made in 351(k) regarding DS qualification.

5.3.1 CLINICAL EFFICACY

The most significant cost element in developing biosimilars is patient efficacy testing. As of the end of 2023, 194 clinical efficacy trials for biosimilars were listed on clinicaltrials.gov, with a total enrollment of 91,760 subjects [40]. The cost per patient is difficult to estimate because of the differences in the complexity of trials. However, a detailed study estimated this at around $54,000 [41]; applying this figure to the currently listed trials in clinicaltrials.gov produces a staggering amount of five billion

Number of Publications

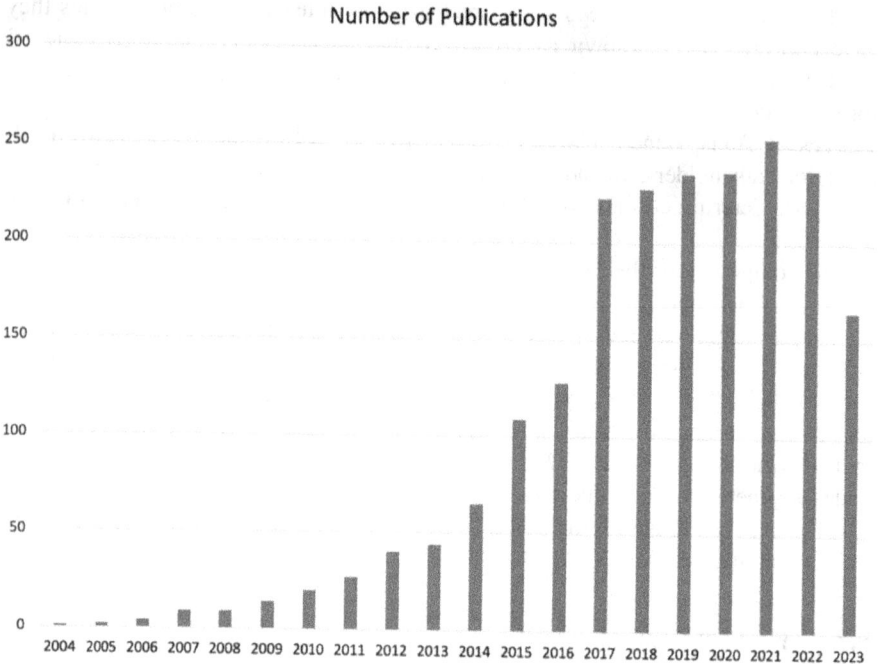

FIGURE 5.2   The number of papers published on the clinical efficacy testing of biosimilars posted in PubMed as of 14 November 2023. (Total 1778.) (https://pubmed.ncbi.nlm.nih.gov/?term=clinical+efficacy+biosimilar&sort=pubdate)

dollars. That study also concluded that "most comparative efficacy trials supporting the FDA approval of biosimilars appeared to be as rigorous as and often larger, longer, and more costly than pivotal trials for new molecular entities" [41].

Numerous publications (Figure 5.2) have analyzed this requirement and reported that these studies cannot fail for scientific and statistical reasons, thus categorizing them as inhumane trials [17]. Removing clinical efficacy testing challenges stakeholders' mindset that testing in patients is the gold standard.

However, one weak point in the BPCIA keeps this mindset holding firm. The BPCIA allows the extrapolation of all indications based on testing in one indication, which the developer can also select. It is well established that the modes of action can differ, and the assumption is that one study if required, is sufficient to ensure the same effectiveness in all indications. For example, biological agents such as tumor necrosis factor inhibitors (etanercept, infliximab, adalimumab, golimumab, and certolizumab pegol) and an interleukin-12/23 inhibitor (ustekinumab) inhibit key inflammatory molecules involved in the pathogenesis of these chronic inflammatory disorders, offering a multifaceted approach to treatment [42]. The differences in the modes of action would demand that if there is a need for efficacy testing, it should extend to all indications. Although well-intentioned, this clause in the BPCIA is a weak element that makes efficacy testing merely a checklist item.

A recent analysis of the EMA biosimilars by its regulators confirms that the efficacy testing was redundant, and products approved based on analytical assessment and clinical pharmacology were proven clinically equivalent [43]. Removing efficacy testing is within the purview of the FDA, and this does not require a legislative change; the FDA would likely be more comfortable with this decision than removing the requirement altogether. The best approach is taken by MHRA, which has amended its guidelines as follows:

> Although each biosimilar development needs to be evaluated on a case-by-case basis, it is considered that, in most cases, a comparative efficacy trial may not be necessary if sound scientific rationale supports this approach. Therefore, a well-argued justification for the absence of an efficacy trial should be appended to CTD Module 1 of the submitted application. [24]

The author conducted an opinion poll on LinkedIn, and the results, although coming from a diversified audience, do not support waiving efficacy testing (Figure 5.3). It is difficult to explain the fine details of the scientific reasons for this lack of support since this is the first time in the history of drug development that we are testing the equivalence of efficacy, including analytical assessment and clinical pharmacology profiling, after establishing the equivalence of the characteristics that determine and demonstrate efficacy. The FDA has excellently educated stakeholders about these subtle considerations [44], yet the challenge of convincing stakeholders remains.

5.3.2 INTERCHANGEABILITY

A recent guideline on labeling biosimilars removes any mention of the biosimilar's interchangeable status from the prescribing information, stating that this status is a legal description rather than a quality classification [46]. This was done in response to repeated questions about the scientific basis for the switching and alternating studies required to secure interchangeable status. The FDA has also waived such testing

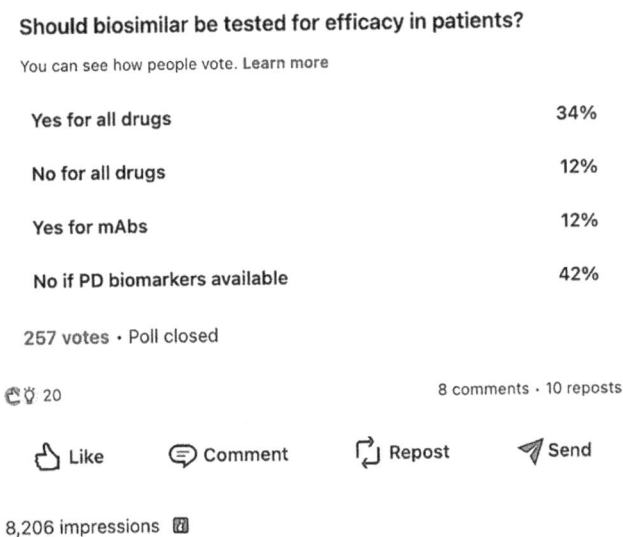

Should biosimilar be tested for efficacy in patients?

You can see how people vote. Learn more

Yes for all drugs	34%
No for all drugs	12%
Yes for mAbs	12%
No if PD biomarkers available	42%

257 votes · Poll closed

♥ 20   8 comments · 10 reposts

👍 Like   💬 Comment   🔁 Repost   ✈ Send

8,206 impressions 🔢

FIGURE 5.3 Survey of LinkedIn respondents for clinical efficacy testing of biosimilars [45].

for at least two products, ranibizumab [47] and ustekinumab [48]. Notably, the inter-changeability status was intended for products that are dispensed at the pharmacy level [49], but there is motivation to secure this status since it grants a 12-month exclusivity period; in addition, the perception that an interchangeable product is superior to biosimilars has brought about many misconceptions regarding biosimilars in the minds of the stakeholders. At the patient and prescriber level, having two classes of biosimilars inevitably creates doubts about their safety.

The MHRA [24] makes it clear that:

> Once authorized, a biosimilar product is considered interchangeable with their RP, which means a prescriber can choose the biosimilar medicine over the RP (or vice versa) and expect to achieve the same therapeutic effect. Likewise, a biosimilar product is considered interchangeable with another biosimilar to the same RP [sic]

The EMA [50] states that,

> A biosimilar is a biological medicine highly similar to another already approved biological medicine (the 'reference medicine'). Interchangeability in this context means that the reference medicine can be replaced by a biosimilar without a patient experiencing any changes in the clinical effect.[sic]

Several studies have confirmed that switching and alternating between a reference product and a biosimilar candidate is redundant [51]. The most robust evidence was recently reported in a research paper by the FDA that confirms in a detailed analysis that these studies do not serve any useful purpose in establishing the safety and efficacy of biosimilars (54). The FDA paper is crucial, as the US Senate is preparing to discuss the Red Tape Elimination Act [52]. It is now anticipated that the interchangeable status will be removed in the US.

5.3.3 Immunogenicity

One concern generally raised in many publications [53] relates to patient immunogenicity testing. All therapeutic proteins can be immunogenic, and the FDA has already established that if an immune response, such as the production of neutralizing antibodies, does not affect the disposition kinetics, then such studies are not necessary [51]. The immunogenicity profile of a biosimilar can be better evaluated in healthy subjects as part of the clinical pharmacology profiling since the patients may have compromised immune function, such as when they are being treated for cancer (85).

5.3.4 Nonclinical Development Stage

Because biosimilars are expensive, developers must create a global strategy that employs a single regulatory dossier to obtain regulatory clearances in several jurisdictions. According to the BPCIA, a biosimilar must be similar to the US licensed originator, a product approved under the Public Health Service Act of 1942, as amended, Sect.—351(a). To complete this regulatory dossier, developers must carry out three-way studies involving a product that is licensed in the US, a product that is not licensed in the US, and a biosimilar candidate.

Although the current BPCIA stipulates that it must be a single product granted under 351(a), selecting a different product necessitates bridging compliance, even if approved using the same dossier. Bridging study policies vary from not requiring a bridging study to requiring many pharmacokinetic–pharmacodynamic (PK–PD) trials. Suppose the proposed reference product satisfies all composition, indication, and route of administration requirements and is approved using "basically" equivalent regulatory dossiers. In that case, the FDA may waive bridging studies under 42 USC 262(k)(2)(A)(ii).

As discussed above, the definition of "biosimilar" needs updating:

a biosimilar has no clinically meaningful difference with a 351(a)-licensed biological product, a non-US biological product approved based on the submission of essentially the same dossier as submitted to the FDA for the under 351(a) licensing, a biosimilar licensed under 351(k), or a biosimilar approved in comparison with a non-US reference product as described above.

Before a biosimilar candidate is administered to humans for testing, it undergoes extensive analytical and functional testing to ensure that its structural and formulation variability is comparable to that of the reference product. Since the analytical assessment is the foundation for establishing biosimilarity, the FDA has proactively suggested comparative testing plans (Figure 5.4) [54]. However, the FDA does not mandate any particular testing plan, the choice of which remains up to the developers. A common misconception in the design of analytical assessment studies comes from mixing orthogonal with repetitive studies; as a result, the number of analytical studies submitted to the FDA has ranged from 20 to 80 [55–57].

The high cost of analytical assessment is attributed to validating testing methods beyond what is required for product release. Most of these methods are not validated

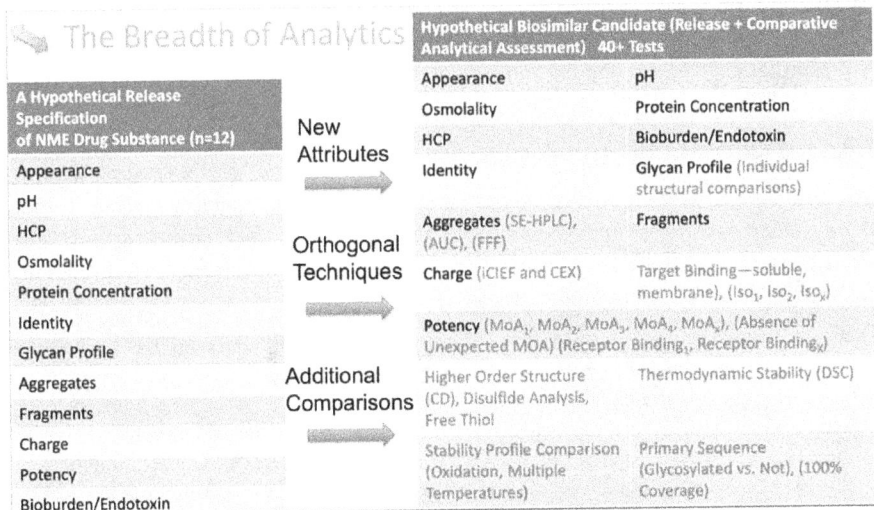

FIGURE 5.4 FDA update on analytical similarity testing protocols to support a claim of biosimilarity [54].

and qualified only as suitable, and the FDA frequently finds compliance with testing product-related attributes to be defective.

Another misconception is that release specification attributes such as protein content and potency are included in comparative testing. While potency testing is confirmed based on receptor binding in functional studies, both attributes have legacy ranges for the approval of injectable products, such as sterility or subvisible particles; the latter should not be confused with aggregates that are not part of legacy attributes. Considering this classification, comparative testing could be reduced significantly. How the statistical modeling of the comparison should be established was the subject of a debate resolved by the FDA in June 2018 when it withdrew the Draft Guidance for Industry: Statistical Approaches to Evaluate Analytical Similarity [58] due to its lack of relevance in comparing critical quality attributes.

Attributes whose limits need tightening are considered impurities. Currently, the limits for biosimilars are as follows: no unmatched impurity, not more than 3% total impurities, no single impurity greater than 1%, and no isoforms, posttranslational modification, or subvisible particles that can affect the safety and efficacy of the product. It is impossible to establish the safety of any of these variations with confidence, and given that the process can be modified to meet these requirements, the FDA should demand compliance with these limits.

If the FDA removes clinical efficacy testing, the 65% cost reduction would leave the period from the development stage to the nonclinical stage, accounting for 65% of the remaining cost. One of the significant hurdles in this field is the availability of reference product samples to test, preferably during the expiry period, to allow a broader variation of attributes. This issue was addressed in the CREATES ACT [59] expediting biosimilar developers' access to reference products; however, this remains a significant issue. Since biosimilar developers may end up with a different remaining shelf life from that of the reference product, release specifications that might differ among biosimilars may be created, raising the question of the interchangeability of biosimilars.

5.3.5 MONOGRAPHS

All these concerns can be resolved, and a substantial cost reduction will be gained if the FDA agrees to reverse its stance on the role of the US Pharmacopeia (USP). The FDA wrote to the USP in May 2018, requesting that it refrain from producing monographs for biological medications [60].

> Because USP's proposed revisions would aggravate existing concerns that a monograph could impede or delay the licensure of biosimilars and other biological products, FDA strongly encourages USP to withdraw its proposal. FDA welcomes future interaction with USP on these issues to ensure that biological product monographs do not create an unnecessary barrier to the availability of biosimilars and other biological products to patients. For example, we see opportunities for optional methodological standards that could encourage innovation and product development.

The FDA was concerned that biologics manufacturers would manipulate the monograph procedure to prevent competition from biosimilars "by incorporating patented characteristics of their product that are not relevant to safety, purity or potency, further impacting competition." This is not a valid argument since the USP would develop the specifications based on FDA guidelines for the analytical assessment of biosimilars. The USP can collect enough batches of the reference products and test them to establish release specifications; validating testing methods will remove the need for side-by-side testing, saving millions of dollars and at least 18 months in developing new biosimilars. The USP can ensure that the test methods do not infringe on any intellectual property and keep updating the release specifications of the reference product if its formulation or presentation changes. However, where the testing methods are not validated, side-by-side testing will still be required, as in the case of primary, secondary, and tertiary structure, potency, and receptor binding.

A detailed study [29] concluded that the time and cost to market can be reduced by more than 20% if product-specific guidelines are available. USP monographs for biosimilars are the most appropriate suggestion to reduce development costs.

5.3.6 DRUG MASTER FILE

The delivery of the biological DS by a third party, following the same paradigm commonly utilized in the production of generic pharmaceuticals, is one viable but seldom-used option. The FDA permits this, but with restrictions [61]:

> Although the FDA's approach to the use of master files in BLAs under the PHS Act largely parallels its approach to the use of DMFs in applications under the Federal Food, Drug, and Cosmetics Act, there is a significant difference: a BLA holder is generally expected to have knowledge of and control over the manufacturing process for the biological product for which it has a license.

As a matter of science, the FDA has traditionally prohibited BLAs under the PHS Act from including information about DSs, intermediates, or DPs by referencing a master file. Instead, the FDA expects such information to be submitted directly within the BLA [62]. Nevertheless, submitting a drug master file (DMF) with information meant for biological product applications is identical to submitting one for chemical generic pharmaceuticals.

If the FDA can establish clear guidelines about using a DS sourced from a third party, it will open the door for many developers who are skilled or financially strong enough to establish DS manufacturing; the area of DPs is still complex for biologicals, but it is readily adopted.

5.3.7 CLINICAL PHARMACOLOGY

The protocol modification for clinical pharmacology testing is another area where development costs can be significantly reduced. Since the purpose of clinical pharmacology testing is to compare, not characterize, the profile, a significant reduction in study size can be achieved by restricting the inclusion criteria to a healthy limited population, such as males between the ages of 25 and 45; another option includes allowing a two-step testing where 10–12 subjects are tested, and if the study power is not met, additional subjects can be added based on the variance in the first study. The data are allowed to be combined. Of the 62 completed pharmacokinetic tests of biosimilars reported on clinicaltrials.gov, the average number of subjects in five trials that enrolled female subjects was 478; 12 studies for males averaged 131 subjects, and all subjects averaged 288 [63]. While these data may not reflect fundamental differences in the population variance, published data on pharmacokinetic studies can calculate smaller study sizes by narrowing down the acceptance criteria.

A comparable PK profile should support PD similarity since the pharmacokinetic profile determines all reactions and their temporal profiles. Biological medications should also function well under the traditional bioequivalence paradigm. The clearance model can also be represented by multicompartmental models, even if single-compartment models are easier to understand. The distribution volume and its rate of change [64,65] are another PK parameter proposed as a measure of the beginning of the action that may be compared to strengthen the validity of PK data.

5.3.8 PD MARKERS

The FDA has approved several products without efficacy testing in patients, provided that these products have comparable PD biomarkers. Examples include erythropoietin and GCSF, discussed in a pivotal paper by the FDA in which studies were conducted to discover new PD biomarkers that could be used to waive clinical efficacy testing [66]. However, a critical analysis of the FDA's conclusions was debated [67] on two grounds: first, according to the FDA, the PD markers need not correlate with clinical efficacy, and second, it is impractical and redundant to expect biosimilar developers to discover new PD biomarkers. The FDA states [68]that,

> PD biomarkers are indicators of a drug's pharmacological effect on its target or targets. For example, the target might be a receptor molecule that initiates a complex signaling cascade. Changes in the levels of proteins along the signaling cascade or modifications to them could be considered pharmacodynamic responses.[sic]
> As such, a correlation between the PD biomarker and clinical outcomes, while beneficial, is not necessary.[sic]

A vital critique of this is that the PD markers may have nonlinear dose-dependent responses; even if the biomarkers are comparable, this does not ensure comparable efficacy, and if the profiles do not match, this does not indicate a lack of equivalent clinical efficacy. Additionally, discovering a new PD biomarker requires extensive scientific studies that include method development and systems validation that go beyond what biosimilar developers can expect. Incidentally, all biological drugs approved by the FDA have already reported biomarkers, and if these are suitable, they can be used instead of discoveries. Briefly, PD biomarkers are irrelevant, except in cases representing a pharmacological response such as erythropoietin, GCSF, and several other cytokines [67].

Clinical efficacy testing is responsible for the majority of the cost of development [2]; however, this cost would be justified if it resolved any query about safety and efficacy. It is well established that once analytical assessment and clinical pharmacology studies have confirmed similarity, clinical efficacy testing does not add value, being the least sensitive of all such studies.

The FDA released guidelines in January 2023 regarding the use of PD indicators to bolster biomarkers' usefulness [69] and the effectiveness of biosimilars. The FDA conducted clinical trials to "find" PD biomarkers; however, these investigations were restricted to proteome testing and failed to distinguish between pharmacology and PD biomarkers [69]. A recent critical analysis of FDA suggestions to discover PD biomarkers for drugs such as monoclonal antibodies that do not usually show any classical PD or pharmacologic markers establishes that PD biomarkers are of little value since there is little correlation with clinical response, as acknowledged by the FDA, leading to the conclusion that regardless of the testing results, the possible nonlinearity of PD responses would make such investigations of little value in ensuring comparable clinical efficacy.

5.3.9 CONTINUOUS SUBMISSION

The 6–8 years development time for biosimilars is partly attributed to repeat studies that can be avoided if the FDA agrees to allow submissions in part at a time. For example, the developer can submit the data on process validation and secure FDA approval of the suitability; the same can be done with analytical assessment reports and clinical pharmacology testing so that when the final BLA is filed, most of the data that is subject to review by the FDA has already been accepted by the FDA. The FDA advises on the data suitability during the development stages to ensure that these studies are acceptable to the FDA in critical stages of submission and the FDA review to avoid a duplicate audit of these data. This view is also supported by the EMA [70].

5.3.10 LABELING

The FDA has proposed changes in the labeling requirements for biosimilars and interchangeable biosimilars in the draft guidance "Labeling for Biosimilar and Interchangeable Biosimilar Products: Guidance for Industry" [46]. When finalized, these nonbinding recommendations will replace previous guidance and questions Q.I.27 and Q.I.28 in the 2020 draft guidance [71]. Under previous draft guidance, the FDA indicated that interchangeable products should include an interchangeability statement on the label. In the September 2023 Federal Register Notice, the FDA explained that "[c]onsistent with [an] evolution in our thinking, the draft guidance states that both biosimilar and interchangeable biosimilar products should contain the same biosimilarity statement in the Highlights of the Prescribing Information."

Furthermore, the draft guidance expands product identification for instances when the reference product labeling describes a clinical study conducted with a non-US-approved biologic. Nevertheless, the biosimilar's labeling should incorporate the same terminology regarding the study's results as the reference products. This identification of the source of the reference product is unnecessary and contradicts the reasons for removing the interchangeable status declaration in the prescribing information on the label. Suppose a product is approved as a biosimilar. In that case, it has met all requirements mandated by the FDA and identifying the products that have used a non-US reference can be part of marketing these products, which can be detrimental to adopting biosimilars.

One significant concession in the new labeling guidance relates to the biosimilar or interchangeable label referring to the pediatric safety data for the reference product and restating and elaborating upon the information using the name of the biosimilar; however, the FDA should clarify that this also means that biosimilars that are not interchangeable need not submit pediatric studies.

5.3.11 SUFFIXES

The FDA has created a unique naming system for biological drugs, wherein a random four-letter suffix is applied to the DS; it also applies to biosimilars, creating a possibility of reference product companies differentiating their product from approved biosimilars. Despite much protest against this requirement, now unique to the US [72], the FDA has continued assigning suffixes to biosimilars and new biologics, even though a globally well-recognized naming system [73] exists. The argument that such a naming system is needed to track the products for postmarket surveillance is invalid since each product has a brand and a National Drug Code assigned [74]. All pharmaceutical products should have a suffix if this coding system is insufficient. Removing suffixes is another step that can be taken to change the mindset of stakeholders that biosimilars are not the same as the reference product; doing so would also allow the RPSs to market their products differently, including their biosimilars.

5.4 THE ROLE OF DEVELOPERS

One way developers can reduce the risk of non-compliance with analytical assessment is to use the same formulation as the reference product, as long as patents do not restrict them. While the primary structure of the biosimilar candidate may match 100%, the secondary and tertiary structures responsible for safety and efficacy can change depending on pH, osmolality, dielectric properties, and other ionic or organic components. Erythropoietin [75] and blood dyscrasia continue to generate safety concerns, even though the current approval system will catch issues before the formulation is approved. Nevertheless, the preference should be to use the exact formulation of the reference product or another approved biosimilar. It is best to avoid the excipient(s) of suggested biosimilar products not utilized in biological products.

Whereas the FDA guidance does not restrict the use of the same cell line type, such as CHO, NS0, Sp2/0, HEK293, and PER.C6, BHK21), *E. coli*, or *S. cerevisiae* used by the reference product, it is well-established that changing the cell line type will produce a different molecule from the reference product, regardless of the optimization of upstream conditions. Developers are thus advised not to use another type of cell line. Additionally, one consideration relates to newer types of high-yielding cell lines that can deliver highly variable products based on the fundamental understanding that pushing the expression system inevitably leads to variance. It is more important to have a cell line yielding consistent expression than one yielding a variable high expression. Notably, higher yields help reduce only the size of the bioreactor, not necessarily the cost of goods that depend on the supply of carbon sources.

Additionally, when a biosimilar candidate is entered, it is compared with a reference product developed more than 20 years ago, including the 12 years of exclusivity;

the high-yielding cell lines are relatively new modifications that require many changes. For example, optimizing the transfection conditions, such as the transfection reagent, DNA concentration, and incubation time, can enhance expression levels; choosing strong and cell-specific promoters can drive the expression of a recombinant protein; using promoters such as CMV or EF1-alpha can generate high-level expression; ensuring that the plasmid or viral vector is designed for high expression may involve codon optimization for the host cell and enhancer elements and the proper selection of expression vectors; optimizing the cell culture media by adjusting nutrient concentrations, pH, and supplements such as serum or growth factors can have a significant impact on expression levels; maintaining the cells at the appropriate temperature and CO_2 levels in the incubator is crucial for optimal protein expression; exploring different transfection methods such as electroporation, lipofection, and viral transduction is done to find the most efficient one for the specific cell line; invoking gene amplification strategies, such as using selectable markers such as dihydrofolate reductase, can increase gene copy number and expression; using transfection enhancers or additives can improve the efficiency of gene delivery and subsequent expression; protein expression levels can be monitored using techniques such as Western blotting or ELISA; and passing cells multiple times can enhance expression [76,77].

It is readily understood that such changes can change the protein structure inherently, so the standard advice is that upgrading the yield of a cell line that yields the desired protein is not advised.

Another way biosimilar developers can reduce their capital expenditures and operational expenditures is to consider a continuous manufacturing process [78] currently recognized by the FDA as an option and provide guidelines for its adoption [78].

Developers can further reduce the cost of manufacturing, testing, and validating three commercial-scale process performance qualification lots by offering to secure approval at a smaller scale and, after the product has been licensed, changing the manufacturing scale using the Q5E guideline [79] that requires analytical comparison of the new batch size with the old ones. This may not be an issue with big pharma, but it can reduce the cost by a few million dollars, which may be significant to smaller developers.

Most biosimilar developers have received multiple complete response letters that delay the approval process significantly. Outsourcing the product-related attribute assessment to qualified contract research organizations is preferred since this testing is not repeated in-house. While the cost can be higher, the overall cost is significantly less if the time lost is considered [80].

5.5   THE ROLE OF THE ASSOCIATIONS

The arrival of biosimilars also brought hundreds of associations supporting biosimilars across the globe. Here, we are analyzing the focus of the US associations and other alliances, particularly the American Biosimilars Council, Association for Accessible Medicines, Biosimilars Forum; Healthcare Distribution Alliance; Biosimilars Council; and Pharmaceutical Research and Manufacturers of America (PhRMA) Biosimilars Committee. The association and alliances like SafeBiologics (https://safebiologics.org/) and associations like the PhRMA Foundation (https://phrma.org/en), Biotechnology Innovation Organization (https://www.bio.org/), both created by the reference product companies promote maintaining extensive testing of biosimilars as a means of slowing down their entry.

Biosimilar use is limited in some healthcare systems because many healthcare professionals and patients do not understand biosimilars well. The knowledge gap is exacerbated by disparagement of biosimilars and dissemination of misinformation, such as statements about biosimilar science or policy that are factually incorrect; misleading information, where the information is correct but is provided out of context; incomplete information, where only partial or a limited set of facts are provided; creation of a false narrative, especially in scientific and medical literature, that provides a set of references to support incorrect conclusions; and negative message framing of factual statements to create a negative perception. The associations of biosimilar developers and other stakeholders can counter disparagement and misinformation about biosimilars. However, the idea of governmental agencies getting involved and providing oversight is unrealistic and impractical, as suggested by some [81]. Proposals that physicians, nurses, pharmacists, and patient advocacy groups should work together to provide patients with consistent, positive messages about the value of biosimilars are of little value.

The only proper way to remove these misconceptions is the efforts of biosimilar associations; however, the focus should not be on educating about biosimilars, for it will fall within the same doctrine used to spread misinformation. Why would anyone trust a biosimilar association more than one representing the reference product companies? The FDA has created a remarkable dossier of education material mandated by the Biosimilars User Fee Amendment (BsUFAIII) funding [82]. The association should only direct the target audience to the FDA or reproduce what the FDA has said. And the most effective tool will be to counteract all misinformation line by line and reference by reference and publicize it. Classic statements of disinformation include such craftily put-together statements [83]:

> Biosimilars are "similar to" but not exact copies of biologics, and small differences can have unexpected or harmful clinical outcomes for patients. While the ultimate goal is to find a balance between producing economical drugs and respecting the drug-discovery process, patient safety should be paramount.
>
> Doctors and patients should be able to carefully choose the best course of treatment rather than have legislators and regulators decide for them.
>
> The interchangeable designation has not only boosted physician and patient confidence, and it has done so without becoming a barrier to biosimilar uptake and savings. In conclusion, weakening the interchangeability standard is an unnecessary and potentially harmful step.

What these opinions fail to state is that the FDA has the right to ask for any number of studies as it deems necessary to ensure safety; it is the exclusivity given to interchangeable products that are at stake as it has a financial impact on the developers who can shell out another 100 million dollars. These statements should have also quoted the FDA that such testing is unnecessary [84–87]. These opinion leaders have no qualification to second-guess the FDA perspective, but these statements have an impact, so the biosimilar associations should confront these attempts as their primary task.

Unfortunately, the biosimilar associations are engaging in an entirely reverse plan; they are saying that using biosimilars will save a lot of money, which is already expected, but it is not the reason to use a biosimilar. The repeated slogans that the US biosimilars have generated $21 Billion in savings in the past 6 years alone fail to tell that the biological drugs still cost hundreds of billions of dollars.

Another misgiving of the biosimilar associations is that they get dragged into misconceived conclusions. For example, all big pharma and their alliances are opposed to the price negotiations allowed under the Inflation Control Act [88]; when biosimilar associations join hands with them, it leads to a loss of confidence in their views, for they cannot agree and disagree with others at the same time.

5.6 CONCLUSIONS

For biosimilars to deliver affordable care, they must first be accessible; today, only 12 molecules out of more than 100 such choices are available in the US. Second, they must be available at a lower cost. To achieve this goal, there is a dire need for all stakeholders to join hands: the US Congress, the FDA, the developers, and their associations. If the actions in this proposal are taken, two significant impacts are anticipated: a substantial reduction in the cost of developing biosimilars that will bring entry of dozens of new biosimilars; the small to midsize companies can afford to sell biosimilars at a much lower cost as well, breaking the pricing barrier significantly, likely to a point where the big pharma will go out of biosimilars business.

Some changes to the BPCIA will require amendments to this bill, such as removing the interchangeable status and amending the patent litigation process, bringing it in concordance with such requirements for other drugs.

However, as the slow process of legislative actions proceeds, the FDA has full authority to bring significant changes, such as allowing interchangeability to the first biosimilar application; this will expedite the entry of newer molecules. However, the FDA cannot remove this designation until it is amended in the BPCIA. The FDA can also eliminate clinical efficacy testing, rationalize analytical assessment, and optimize clinical pharmacology testing, all of which have a major impact on the entry of new biosimilars. Other actions by the FDA, such as allowing DMF filings, allowing reference products for other biosimilars, and eliminating bridging studies, could also substantially reduce the cost. Letting the USP create monographs would bring in hundreds of new applications in a short time. The FDA should also adopt an ongoing filing system to ensure faster development.

The role of developers is also essential. For example, requesting the FDA to allow the use of DS from a third party and challenging the FDA at an interesting point: "if residual uncertainty remains, additional clinical studies may be required." The FDA should identify the "residual uncertainty" after analytical and clinical pharmacology assessment and also tell that a given clinical study will remove this uncertainty. The developers will find that the FDA will be willing to waive any additional testing in patients; the "clinical studies" could be another PK study or *in silico* analysis—the options that the developers had not exploited. Notably, the FDA recently issued a new guideline, Generally Accepted Scientific Knowledge [89] that encourages developers to bring scientific challenges to their development plans. Similarly, the arrival of Artificial Intelligence and Machine Learning should be considered in designing the testing protocols to achieve maximum efficiency [32].

The developers can also outsource the development work while they establish in-house manufacturing, and after the biosimilar has been approved, transfer the technology under the Q5E legislation, wherein the products manufactured are compared with prior batches and mostly in analytical testing. This approach will reduce the burden of delayed approval from the findings of the FDA audits, which can be avoided by filing based on a CDMO work and then transferring it under Q5E.

Finally, the associations financially supported by biosimilar developers need to create a constructive strategy focusing on abetting the misinformation about biosimilars, not educating about biosimilar as this should be left to the FDA. These associations and alliances also should not get dragged into debates where they are not competent since their counterparts are much smarter with enormous funding.

The development cost can be reduced to approximately $10–20 million. At this level, scores of smaller-scale developers can be expected to enter the market, bringing in the 100+ biologicals ready for entry as biosimilars. While the cost calculations presented above are based on hands-on experience, these costs can vary significantly depending on the nature of the molecule; however, the cost of goods of biological drugs has been ascertained; the World Health Organization has calculated that monoclonal antibodies cost $95–200/ g [90] that is still considered too high to bring these drugs to patients across the globe. The FDA has taken several steps to reduce development costs, such as releasing the first continuous manufacturing guidelines for biological drugs. This practice can substantially reduce capital expenditure and the cost of goods [89].

Finally, the suggestions made above, the author anticipates, will be subject to criticism, and this is a normal phase of transition of any technology; the history of humanity is filled with such changes, albeit when financial vested interests are involved in keeping the development cost high, these can take a longer time to be accepted.

REFERENCES

1. Pfizer. Biosimilars. https://www.pfizerbiosimilars.com/biosimilars-development#:~:text= The%20development%20of%20a%20biosimilar,approximately%20two%20years%20to% 20develop2023.
2. McKinsey. Three imperatives for R&D in biosimilars. https://www.mckinsey.com/ industries/life-sciences/our-insights/three-imperatives-for-r-and-d-in-biosimilars.
3. Francis Ta. Biosimilars. https://www.tandfonline.com/doi/full/10.1080/14712598. 2021.1849132#:~:text=The%20lower%20price%20of%20biosimilars,4%2C%20Citation %2024%2C%20Citation%20252021.
4. Kvien, T.K.; Patel, K.; Strand, V. The cost savings of biosimilars can help increase patient access and lift the financial burden of health care systems. *Semin. Arthritis Rheum.* 2022, 52, 151939.
5. Drugs I. US Approved Proteins. https://drugs.ncats.io/substances?facet=Development %20Status%2FUS%20Approved%20Rx&facet=Highest%20Phase%2FApproved &facet=Substance%20Class%2Fprotein&facet=Substance%20Form%2FPrincipal %20Form&page=1.

6. Watch BM. Overview of the "Patent Dance" under the Biologics Price Competition and Innovation Act https://www.bigmoleculewatch.com/wp-content/uploads/sites/2/2022/12/Patent-Dance-Guide-December-2022.pdf.

7. Mckinsey R&D Biosimilars. https://www.mckinsey.com/industries/life-sciences/our-insights/three-imperatives-for-r-and-d-in-biosimilars.

8. Gupta, R.; Shah, N.D.; Ross, J.S. Generic drugs in the United States: Policies to address pricing and competition. *Clin. Pharmacol. Ther.* 2019, 105(2), 329–337.

9. Borchers, A.T.; Hagie, F., Keen, C.L.; Gershwin, M.E. The history and contemporary challenges of the US Food and Drug Administration. *Clin. Ther.* 2007, 29(1), 1–16.

10. Congress U. Title VII-Improving Access to Innovative Medical Therapies Subtitle A-Biologics Price Competition and Innovation. https://www.fda.gov/media/78946/download.

11. Kennedy. Biologics Price Competition and Innovation Act of 2007. https://www.congress.gov/bill/110th-congress/senate-bill/16952007.

12. Congress U. SEC. 7001. <<NOTE: 42 USC 201 note>>. https://www.congress.gov/bill/111th-congress/house-bill/3590/text?s=4&r=26&q=%7B%22search%22%3A%22biosimilar%22%7D.

13. Public Law 111-148—Patient Protection and Affordable Care Act. https://www.govinfo.gov/app/details/PLAW- 111publ148.

14. Congress U. 21 USC Ch. 9: FEDERAL FOOD, DRUG, AND COSMETIC ACT https://uscode.house.gov/view.xhtml?path=/prelim@title21/chapter9&edition=prelim.

15. Waxman H. H.R.6257—Access to Life-Saving Medicine Act. https://www.congress.gov/bill/109th-congress/house-bill/6257/text?s=3&r=1&q=%7B%22search%22%3A%22H.R.+6257+109th+Congress%22%7D2006.

16. Public Health Service Act, 1944. Public Health Rep. 1994;109(4):468.

17. Niazi, S. Scientific rationale for waiving clinical efficacy testing of biosimilars. *Drug Des. Dev. Ther.* 2022, 16, 2803–2815.

18. Waxman H. H.R.1038—Access to Life-Saving Medicine Act. https://www.congress.gov/bill/110th-congress/house-bill/1038?q=%7B%22search%22%3A%22waxman+1038%22%7D&s=5&r=1.

19. Inslee. H.R. 1956 (IH) —Patient Protection and Innovative Biologic Medicines Act of 2007. https://www.govinfo.gov/app/details/BILLS-110hr1956ih.

20. Gregg. S. 1505 (IS) —Affordable Biologics for Consumers Act. https://www.congress.gov/bill/110th-congress/house-bill/1956.

21. Guidelines relevant for advanced therapy medicinal products. https://www.ema.europa.eu/en/human-regulatory/research-development/advanced-therapies/guidelines-relevant-advanced-therapy-medicinal-products.

22. Congress U. FDA Modernization Act 2.0. https://www.congress.gov/bill/117th-congress/senate-bill/5002.

23. Niazi, S.K. End animal testing for biosimilar approval. *Science* 2022, 377(6602), 162–163.

24. MHRA. Guidance on the licensing of biosimilar products. https://www.gov.uk/government/publications/guidance-on-the-licensing-of-biosimilar-products/guidance-on-the-licensing-of-biosimilar-products.

25. Nagai, S. Current situation of oncology biosimilars in Japan. *Lancet Oncol.* 2021, 22(3), e82.

26. Rathore, A.S.; Stevenson, J.G.; Chhabra, H.; Maharana, C. The global landscape on interchangeability of biosimilars. *Expert Opin. Biol. Ther.* 2022;22(2):133–148.

27. Congress U. Bills Related to Biosimilars. https://www.congress.gov/search?q=%7B%22search%22%3A%5B%22Biosimilars%22%5D%2C%22type%22%3A%22bills%22%2C%22bill-status%22%3A%5B%22law%22%5D%7D.

28. Congress U. Biosimilar Laws Approved https://www.congress.gov/search?q=%7B%22search%22%3A%5B%22Biosimilars+patent%22%5D%2C%22type%22%3A%22bills%22%2C%22bill-status%22%3A%22law%22%7D.

29. HHS/ ERG. Task order no. HHSP23337005T; Contract no. HHSP233201500055I; Cost of generic drug development and approval. https://aspe.hhs.gov/sites/default/files/documents/20e14b66420440b9e726c61d281cc5a5/cost-of-generic-drugs-erg.pdf.

30. Hasson, K.M., Salgado, M. Biosimilars Enter the Courts: How Will Patent Infringement Settlements Be Tested for Validity Under Antitrust Laws? https://www.pillsburylaw.com/images/content/1/0/109239.pdf

31. Niazi, S.K.; Mariam, Z. Reinventing therapeutic proteins: Mining a treasure of new therapies. *Biologics* 2023, 3(2), 72–94.

32. Niazi, S.K. The coming of age of AI/ML in drug discovery, development, clinical testing, and manufacturing: The FDA perspectives. *Drug Des. Dev. Ther.* 2023, 17, 2691–2725.

33. López-Astorga, M.; Ragni, M.; Johnson-Laird, P.N. The probability of conditionals: A review. *Psychon. Bull. Rev.* 2022, 29(1), 1–20.

34. Wong, T.T.-Y.; Morsanyi, K. The link between transitive reasoning and mathematics achievement in preadolescence: the role of relational processing and deductive reasoning. *Think. Reason.* 2023, 29(4), 531–558.

35. Lange, M. Transitivity, self-explanation, and the explanatory circularity argument against Humean accounts of natural law. *Synthese.* 2018, 195(3), 1337–1353.

36. Böhm, A.K.; Steiner, I.M.; Stargardt, T. Market diffusion of biosimilars in off-patent biologic drug markets across Europe. *Health Policy* 2023, 132, 104818.

37. Gale, A. If pharmacy benefit managers raise drug prices, then why are they needed? *Mo Med.* 2023, 120(4), 243–244.

38. Ph RMA. It's PBMs, not patents, blocking competition. https://phrma.org/Blog/Its-PBMs-not-patents-blocking-competition.

39. Congress U. Pharmacy Benefits Manager. https://www.congress.gov/search?q=%7B%22congress%22%3A%5B%22118%22%5D%2C%22source%22%3A%22all%22%2C%22search%22%3A%22pharmacy%20benefits%20managers%22%7D.

40. Niazi S. Scientific rationale for waiving clinical efficacy testing of biosimilars. *Drug Des Devel Ther.* 2022,16, 2803–2815. doi: 10.2147/DDDT.S378813..

41. Moore, T.J.; Mouslim, M.C.; Blunt, J.L.; Alexander, G.C.; Shermock, K.M. Assessment of availability, clinical testing, and US food and drug administration review of biosimilar biologic products. *JAMA Int. Med.* 2021, 181(1), 52–60.

42. Brezinski, E.A.; Armstrong, A.W. An evidence-based review of the mechanism of action, efficacy, and safety of biologic therapies in the treatment of psoriasis and psoriatic arthritis. *Curr. Med. Chem.* 2015, 22(16), 1930–1942.

43. Kirsch-Stefan, N.; Guillen, E.; Ekman, N.; Barry, S.; Knippel, V.; Killalea, S.; et al. Do the outcomes of clinical efficacy trials matter in regulatory decision-making for biosimilars? *BioDrugs* 2023, 37(6), 855–871.

44. FDA. Multimedia Educational Materials for Biosimilars. https://www.fda.gov/drugs/biosimilars/multimedia-education-materials-biosimilars.

45. Niazi, S. Should biosimilars be tested for efficacy in patients? https://www.linkedin.com/feed/update/urn:li:activity:7129824642021670912/?commentUrn=urn%3Ali%3Acomment%3A(ugcPost%3A7129824640956301312%2C7129871966966034432)&dashCommentUrn=urn%3Ali%3Afsd_comment%3A(7129871966966034432%2Curn%3Ali%3AugcPost%3A7129824640956301312)&dashReplyUrn=urn%3Ali%3Afsd_comment%3A(7129883094685274112%2Curn%3Ali%3AugcPost%3A7129824640956301312)&replyUrn=urn%3Ali%3Acomment%3A(ugcPost%3A7129824640956301312%2C7129883094685274112)2023.

46. FDA. Labeling for Biosimilar and Interchangeable Biosimilar Products Guidance for Industry. https://www.fda.gov/regulatory-information/search-fda-guidance-documents/labeling-biosimilar-and-interchangeable-biosimilar-products.

47. FDA. Cimerli: ranibizumab-eqrn. https://www.accessdata.fda.gov/drugsatfda_docs/label/2022/761165s000lbl.pdf.

48. FDA. Wezlana (ustekinumab-auub). https://www.accessdata.fda.gov/drugsatfda_docs/label/2023/761285s000,761331s000lbl.pdf: FDA; 2023.

49. Niazi, S.K. No two classes of biosimilars: Urgent advice to the US Congress and the FDA. *J. Clin. Pharm. Ther.* 2022, 47(9), 1352–1361.

50. Agency EM. Biosimilar medicines can be interchanged. https://www.ema.europa.eu/en/news/biosimilar-medicines-can-be-interchanged#:~:text=A%20biosimilar%20is%20a%20biological, changes%20in%20the%20clinical%20effect.2022.

51. Barbier, L.; Ebbers, H.C.; Declerck, P.; Simoens, S.; Vulto, A.G.; Huys, I. The efficacy, safety, and immunogenicity of switching between reference biopharmaceuticals and biosimilars: A systematic review. *Clin. Pharmacol. Ther.* 2020, 108(4), 734–755.

52. Congress U. S.2305—Biosimilar Red Tape Elimination Act. https://www.congress.gov/bill/118th-congress/senate-bill/2305?q=%7B%22search%22%3A%22Interchangeability%22%7D&s=5&r=42023.

53. Heron, C.E.; Ghamrawi, R.I.; Balogh, E.A.; Feldman, S.R. Immunogenicity of biologic and biosimilar therapies for psoriasis and impact of novel immunoassays for immunogenicity detection. *Am. J. Clin. Dermatol.* 2021, 22(2), 221–231.

54. Welch, J. FDA: A Firm Foundation—The Power of Analytics in Biosimilar Development. https://www.fda.gov/media/163283/download.

55. FDA. Bevacizumab (Amgen): 761028Orig1s000 PRODUCT QUALITY REVIEW(S) https://www.accessdata.fda.gov/drugsatfda_docs/nda/2017/761028Orig1s000SumR.pdf.

56. FDA. Cyltezo: FDA Filing Chemistry Review. https://www.accessdata.fda.gov/drugsatfda_docs/nda/2017/761058Orig1s000ClinPharmR.pdf.

57. FDA. Abrilada; 761118Orig1s000. PRODUCT QUALITY REVIEW(S). https://www.accessdata.fda.gov/drugsatfda_docs/nda/2019/761118Orig1s000ChemR.pdf.

58. FDA Withdraws Draft Guidance for Industry: Statistical Approaches to Evaluate Analytical Similarity. https://www.fda.gov/drugs/drug-safety-and-availability/fda-withdraws-draft-guidance-industry-statistical-approaches-evaluate-analytical-similarity#:~:text=After%20considering%20public%20comments%20that, could%20impact%20the%20cost%20and: FDA.

59. FDA. How To Obtain a Covered Product Authorization. https://www.fda.gov/regulatory-information/search-fda-guidance-documents/how-obtain-covered-product-authorization.

60. FDA. FDA Letter to USP Re_Drug Product Monographs for Biological Products. https://www.fda.gov/media/112103/download.

61. FDA. Drug Master File. https://www.fda.gov/media/131861/download.

62. FDA. Licensed Biological Products with Supporting Documents. https://www.fda.gov/vaccines-blood-biologics/licensed-biological-products-supporting-documents.

63. ClinicalTrials. Completed pharmacokinetic studies of biosimilars. https://clinicaltrials.gov/search?term=biosimilar&intr=pharmacokinetics&aggFilters=status:com.

64. Niazi, S. Volume of distribution as a function of time. *J. Pharm. Sci.* 1976, 65(3), 452–454.

65. Wesolowski, C.A.; Wesolowski, M.J.; Babyn, P.S.; Wanasundara, S.N. Time varying apparent volume of distribution and drug half-lives following intravenous bolus injections. *PLoS One* 2016, 11(7), e0158798.

66. Chiu, K.; Racz, R.; Burkhart, K.; Florian, J.; Ford, K.; Iveth Garcia, M.; et al. New science, drug regulation, and emergent public health issues: The work of FDA's division of applied regulatory science. *Front. Med. (Lausanne)* 2022, 9, 1109541.

67. Niazi, S.K. A critical analysis of the FDA's omics-driven pharmacodynamic biomarkers to establish biosimilarity. *Pharmaceuticals (Basel)* 2023, 16, 1556.

68. FDA. The Role of Pharmacodynamic Biomarkers in Biosimilar Drug Development. https://www.fda.gov/drugs/cder-small-business-industry-assistance-sbia/role-pharmacodynamic-biomarkers-biosimilar-drug-development#:~:text=PD%20biomarkers%20are%20indicators%20of, could%20be%20considered%20pharmacodynamic%20responses.2023.

69. Florian, J.; Sun, Q.; Schrieber, S.J.; White, R.; Shubow, S.; Johnson-Williams, B.E.; et al. Pharmacodynamic biomarkers for biosimilar development and approval: A workshop summary. *Clin. Pharmacol. Ther.* 2023, 113(5), 1030–1035.

70. Kurki, P.; Kang, H.N.; Ekman, N.; Knezevic, I.; Weise, M.; Wolff-Holz, E. Regulatory evaluation of biosimilars: Refinement of principles based on the scientific evidence and clinical experience. *BioDrugs* 2022, 36(3), 359–371.

71. FDA. Biosimilarity and Interchangeability: Additional Draft Q&As on Biosimilar Development and the BPCI Act Guidance for Industry. https://www.fda.gov/regulatory-information/search-fda-guidance-documents/biosimilarity-and-interchangeability-additional-draft-qas-biosimilar-development-and-bpci-act.

72. FDA. Citizen Petition from University of Illinois, College of Pharmacy. https://www.regulations.gov/document/FDA-2023-P-3766-0001.

73. WHO. INN for biological and biotechnological substances. https://www.who.int/teams/health-product-and-policy-standards/inn/inn-bio/inn-bio-inn.

74. FDA. National Drug Code Database Background Information. https://www.fda.gov/drugs/development-approval-process-drugs/national-drug-code-database-background-information#:~:text=2.-, NDC%20Number, is%20assigned%20by%20the%20FDA.

75. Abraham, I.; MacDonald, K. Clinical safety of biosimilar recombinant human erythropoietins. *Expert. Opin. Drug Saf.* 2012, 11(5), 819–840.

76. Xiao, S.; Shiloach, J.; Betenbaugh, M.J. Engineering cells to improve protein expression. *Curr. Opin. Struct. Biol.* 2014, 26, 32–38.

77. Foreman, R.; Wollman, R. Mammalian gene expression variability is explained by underlying cell state. *Mol. Syst. Biol.* 2020, 16(2), e9146.

78. National Academies of Sciences Engineering, and Medicine, Division on Earth and Life Studies, Board on Chemical Sciences and Technology. *Continuous Manufacturing for the Modernization of Pharmaceutical Production: Proceedings of a Workshop.* Washington (DC): National Academies Press (US) Copyright 2019 by the National Academy of Sciences. All rights reserved; 2019.

79. FDA. Q5E Comparability of Biotechnological/Biological Products Subject to Changes in Their Manufacturing Process. https://www.fda.gov/media/71489/download.

80. Niazi, S. BioRationality: A Dr Sarfaraz Niazi Column-Avoid Delays in Biosimilar Approvals Due to CRLs. https://www.centerforbiosimilars.com/view/biorationality-a-dr-sarfaraz-niazi-column-avoid-delays-in-biosimilar-approvals-due-to-crls:Centerfor Biosimilars; 2023.

81. Cohen, H.P.; McCabe, D. The importance of countering biosimilar disparagement and misinformation. *BioDrugs* 2020, 34(4), 407–414.

82. FDA. Biosimilar Program Updates and What's New Under BsUFA III. https://www.fda.gov/media/170937/download.

83. Alliance S. Biologic Safety. https://safebiologics.org/biologic-safety/2023.

84. Park, J.P.; Jung, B.; Park, H.K.; Shin, D.; Jung, J.A.; Ghil, J.; et al. Interchangeability for biologics is a legal distinction in the USA, not a clinical one. *BioDrugs* 2022, 36(4), 431–436.

85. Dong, X.; Tsong, Y. Equivalence assessment for interchangeability based on two-sided tests. *J. Biopharm. Stat.* 2014, 24(6), 1312–1331.

86. Druedahl, L.C.; Kälvemark Sporrong, S.; Minssen, T.; Hoogland, H.; De Bruin, M.L.; van de Weert, M.; Almarsdóttir, A.B. Interchangeability of biosimilars: A study of expert views and visions regarding the science and substitution. *PLoS One* 2022, 17(1), e0262537.

87. Lasala, R.; Abrate, P.; Zovi, A.; Santoleri, F. Safety and Effectiveness of Multiple Switching Between Originators and Biosimilars: Literature Review and Status Report on Interchangeability. *Ther. Innov. Regul. Sci.* 2023, 57(2), 352–364.

88. Niazi, S.K. The inflation reduction act: A boon for the generic and biosimilar industry. *J. Clin. Pharm. Ther.* 2022, 47(11), 1738–1751.

89. Niazi, S.K. The FDA's new guideline "Generally Accepted Scientific Knowledge" (GASK): An opportunity to expedite the approval of biosimilars. *Pharmaceuticals (Basel).* 2023, 16(11), 517.

90. World Health Organization. Regional Office for Europe. Call for consultant on monoclonal antibodies for infectious diseases. https://www.who.int/news-room/articles-detail/call-for-consultant-on-monoclonal-antibodies-for-infectious-diseases2021.

6 Repurposing Biosimilars

6.1 INTRODUCTION

The famous quote of the 1988 Nobel Laureate in Medicine, James Black [1], that 'the best way to discover a new drug is to start with an old one,' sets the theme of reinventing therapeutic proteins to capitalize on their multibillion-dollar cost. Fourteen years from their development [2] is a novel approach to introduce biological therapies based on approved therapeutic proteins' safety and efficacy claims. It could be a new dose, a new delivery system, a new route of administration, a new indication, or a new combination with other therapeutic proteins, chemical drugs, or radiation sources.

These reinventing options are widely adopted [3]—mainly when treating rare and neglected diseases with limited patients. However, reinventing also helps in situations where faster development is critical, as happened during the COVID-19 or Ebola outbreaks which led to a vigorous push to repurpose the use of multiple antibodies, as there was no time to wait for a new drug.

The main advantage of the reinventing strategy is that its safety and manufacturing processes are already established, which reduces the need for extensive research and development, including preclinical testing, thus, taking the reinvented entity directly to phase III testing in most cases [4]. This is a major cost saving, allowing a continued amortization of the initial development cost.

Drug reinventing often arrives serendipitously from the surprising effects observed for an approved drug. As 'chance favors only the prepared mind [5], serendipity has produced significant advances in the history of medicine and selective optimization of side activities of drug molecules for generating new drugs' [6]. Examples of chemical drugs have been repurposed for benign prostatic hyperplasia, angina, sedation, nausea, and insomnia; later, they were repurposed for use in hair loss, erectile dysfunction, and leprosy, respectively [7]. Examples of serendipitous discovery include sildenafil, intended for the treatment of hypertension and ended up as the most popular male erectile dysfunction treatment; dimethyl fumarate, developed to treat multiple sclerosis [8], ended up treating psoriasis [9]; or the antiviral drug remdesivir under testing to treat Ebola infection, ended up treating COVID-19 [10].

Beyond serendipity, we can reinvent new drugs using technologies such as drug–target interactions (DTIs). AI-driven in silico tools significantly helps DTI mapping for drug reinvention. This technique has played a vital role in identifying potential therapeutics during the COVID-19 pandemic. A deep learning (DL) model trained on DTI, molecule transformer–drug–target interaction (MT-DTI), has uncovered alternate uses of available drugs: atazanavir and remdesivir efavirenz, ritonavir, and dolutegravir as inhibitors against SARS-CoV-2 protein [11]. CATNIP, a machine learning (ML) model for drug repurposing, uses similarity data of the molecules based on their structure, target, and pathway information for drug reinvention [12].

DOI: 10.1201/9781003404637-6

Besides identifying clinical targets, AI-based models can also identify adverse effects of therapeutics. For instance, chemical fingerprint data were used to develop a model which predicted that 22 FDA-approved drugs have potential contributions to heart failure. Later, experimental validation confirmed that 8 out of 22 anticipated therapeutics had cardioprotective activities [13].

A newer [14] approach for drug repurposing involves two-stage prediction and ML. First, diseases are clustered by gene expression because similar altered gene expression patterns imply critical pathways shared in different disease conditions. Next, drug efficacy is assessed by the reversibility of abnormal gene expression, and results are clustered to identify repurposing targets. Finally, the functions of affected genes are analyzed to examine consistency with expected drug efficacy.

Adding a new indication is one of the fastest routes to reinventing therapeutic proteins because of the diversity of pharmacologic responses of therapeutic proteins; they need to be discovered. It is anticipated that new indications can be added to most approved therapeutic proteins, opening a vast treasure of therapies at a much-reduced development cost since the therapeutic protein's safety is already established. Examples of therapeutic proteins that have received new indications recently include Actemra (tocilizumab), Adcetris (brentuximab vedotin), Dupixent (dupilumab), Enhertu (fam-trastuzumab deruxtecan-nxki), Eylea (aflibercept), Hadlima (adalimumab-bwwd), Imfinzi (durvalumab), Jemperli (dostarlimab-gxly), Kevzara (sarilumab), Keytruda (pembrolizumab), Libtayo (cemiplimab-rwlc), Takhzyro (lanadelumab-flyo), Tecentriq (atezolizumab), Tezspire (tezepelumab-ekko), Trodelvy (sacituzumab govitecan-hziy), and Trogarzo (ibalizumab-uiyk) [15]. A biosimilar can also obtain a new indication if not protected by a patent, which significantly expands the drug's utility.

6.2 UNDERSTANDING THERAPEUTIC PROTEINS

"Therapeutic protein" refers to recombinant DNA (rDNA) products that join DNA from different species and subsequently insert the hybrid DNA into a host cell, often a bacterium or mammalian cell, to express the target protein. UC San Francisco and Stanford researchers created this molecular chimera in 1972 [16]. Stanley Cohen of Stanford and Herbert Boyer of UCSF received the US patent in 1980. On 26 July 1974, ten researchers, including six future Nobel Laureates (James Watson, Paul Berg, Stanley Cohen, David Baltimore, Ronald Davis, and Daniel Nathans), wrote a letter in Science [17] urging that the NIH regulate recombinant DNA technology.

The first rDNA product came in 1982 when the rDNA insulin was approved [18]; now, hundreds of recombinant proteins are approved by regulatory agencies [19]. Examples of this diverse class of compounds include interferons, cytokines, interleukins, thrombocytes, growth factors, coagulation factors, blood factors, anticoagulants, Fc fusion proteins, monoclonal antibodies (mAbs), etc. [20]. The global biologics market size is expected to reach around USD 719.94 billion by 2030, valued at USD 366.50 billion in 2021 and growing at a CAGR of 7.15% from 2022 to 2030. The current market of therapeutic proteins exceeds USD 380 billion [21].

Therapeutic proteins replace a protein that is abnormal or deficient in a particular disease or augment the body's supply of a beneficial protein to help reduce the impact of disease or chemotherapy. Genetically engineered proteins can closely resemble the natural proteins they replace or be enhanced by adding sugars or other molecules that extend the protein's duration of activity.

For regulatory approval, the FDA treats alpha amino acid polymer with 40 or fewer amino acids as a peptide, not a protein [22]. It is regulated as a drug under the FD&C Act rather than the Public Health Service Act which controls biological drugs. Other definitions of peptide define the range of amino acids from 2 to 50 [23].

The unique properties of proteins arrive from the long chain of amino acids in therapeutic proteins that fold into a three-dimensional (3D) structure of domains that attach to receptors, resulting in pharmacological responses that can be extended to the toxicological response. In addition, proteins are, by nature, immunogenic, a property that can also be modulated by altering the structure.

Polypeptide chains are combinations of 20 different types of amino acids resulting in the production of numerous proteins due to the high degree of freedom, as pointed out by Cyrus Levinthal in 1969. Suppose we account for only three states of each bond for an amino acid sequence with 101 residues, 100 peptide bonds, and 199 distinct phi and psi bond angles, in that case, a protein can fold into a maximum of $3,100 = 5 \times 1,047$ possible conformations. It will take approximately 1,027 years to test all the possibilities at a protein sampling rate of $3 \times 1,020$ per year [24,25]. This paradox of the natural folding of proteins was only recently resolved, claiming that as proteins fold into native states, they mostly reach a state of minimum energy and maximum stability. This observation will lead to the use of AI-based protein structure prediction and its confidence in repeatability. This will become a critical exercise in evaluating the safety of copies of proteins as biosimilars, as discussed below.

The high flexibility, structural plasticity, and specificity of intrinsically dynamic systems determine receptor binding modes, pharmacokinetics (PK), pharmacodynamics (PD), bioavailability, drug target, and anti-target protein interactions, and their relative affinity [26]. Briefly, the possible structural diversity of domains suggests that a protein molecule could have multiple modes of action and, thus, therapeutic applications (Figure 6.1).

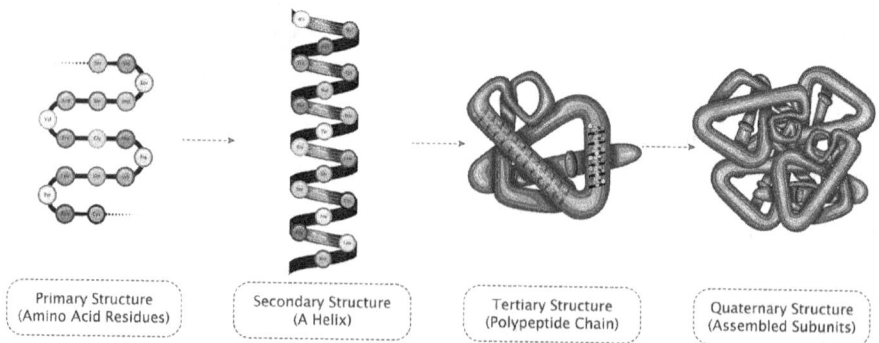

| Primary Structure (Amino Acid Residues) | Secondary Structure (A Helix) | Tertiary Structure (Polypeptide Chain) | Quaternary Structure (Assembled Subunits) |

FIGURE 6.1   Amino acid chains form a secondary structure (helix), resulting in a polypeptide chain folding to form proteins. Licensed from Shutterstock.

The 3D structure of proteins defines their functions; specific domains interact with receptors, triggering pharmacological and toxicological responses. The biological assay reflects the known mechanism and thus serves as a link to clinical activity. Therefore, using relevant biological assay(s) of appropriate precision, accuracy, and sensitivity is essential to confirming no significant functional difference.

A key element of protein structure is the domain resulting from its stable structure that can fold and undergo folding without reference to the rest of the amino acid chain. Domains are not necessarily unique; the same gene can be found in many molecules. The binding domain binds to a specific atom or molecule, such as calcium or DNA. Proteins may have a conformational change as a result of binding. Many proteins depend on their binding domains to work correctly. They are necessary because they aid in the splicing, assembling, and translating proteins [27] (Figure 6.2).

Given the many possible domains, the approved indications of a protein drug only represent a limited activity of the tested or known domains, allowing the discovery of numerous other efficacy profiles. For example, many antibodies were proposed with new indications to control COVID-19 infection [28], and bevacizumab continues to add drug combinations and newer indications in treating age-related macular degeneration [29,30].

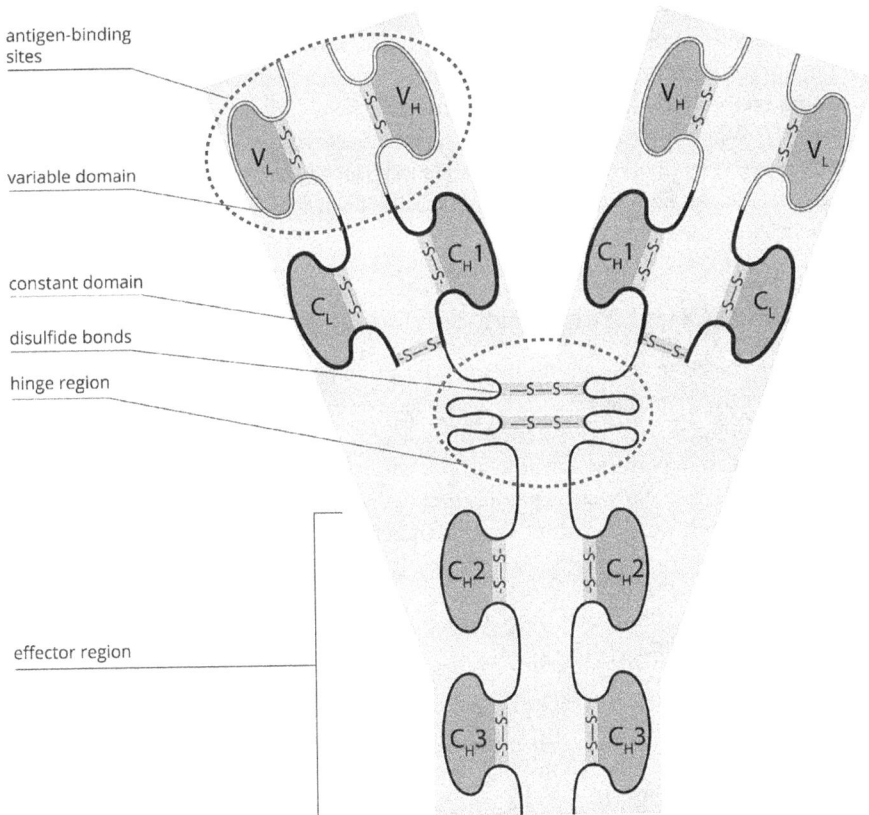

FIGURE 6.2 Variable and constant antibody domains. Licensed from Shutterstock.

mAbs are immunoglobulins that bind to specific protein epitope targets, cancer, and stromal cells, giving them therapeutic properties. The mAb properties of importance are (i) binding affinity to the target antigen; (ii) binding to Fc receptors such as FcγRI, Ia, IIa, IIb, IIIa, IIIb, and FcγRN; (iii) assessment of effector functions such as ADCC and (iv) CDC; (v) molecule characteristics such as charge, pI, hydrophobicity, and glycosylation; and (vi) off-target binding using in silico or in vitro methods such as baculovirus ELISA tools [31,32]. More specifically, for TNFα blockers: C1q, CDC, induction of regulatory macrophage, inhibition of T-cell proliferation, LTα, Mixed Lymphocyte Reaction (MLR), mTNFα, off-target cytokines, reverse signaling, sTNFα, suppression of cytokine secretion, tmTNF-α.

6.3   REINVENTION SCOPE

Advancements in recombinant technology have enabled developers to fine-tune and increase the therapeutic potential of proteins by targeting their structure and function to enhance their disposition half-life, product yield, and purity [33]. Modifying disposition kinetics is also an excellent opportunity to reduce the dosing frequency.

The current reinventing approaches are less serendipitous and more based on rational and systematic approaches; libraries of approved compounds are available from many commercial sources. In addition, several computational and high-content screening methods are currently used to discover new indications for existing molecules [34]. When a hit emerges from a drug reinventing strategy, it can be taken directly into the last phases of clinical trials [35]. However, the side effects of therapeutic proteins can be disease dependent, unlike chemical drugs, requiring creative approaches to establish safety [36].

6.4   INTELLECTUAL PROPERTY

A major hindrance in reinventing therapeutic proteins is their intellectual property protection for the gene that expresses the molecule. If a new indication is patented, it will be allowed once the gene patent expires. However, this bar is coming down fast as many therapeutic proteins are now off the patent [37]. In addition, the intellectual property hurdles go beyond gene patents and include process-related patents that can extend the research work to remove any infringement [38].

6.5   ARTIFICIAL INTELLIGENCE (AI) AND
MACHINE LEARNING (ML)

ML uses algorithms that can recognize patterns within a data set that has been further classified. A subfield of ML is DL, which engages artificial neural networks (ANNs). These comprise a set of "perceptrons," interconnected sophisticated computing elements mimicking biological neurons with their electrical impulses in the brain [39]. ANNs constitute a set of nodes, each receiving a separate input, ultimately converting them to single or multi-linked outputs using algorithms to solve problems. ANNs involve various types, including multilayer perceptron (MLP) networks, recurrent neural networks (RNNs), and convolutional neural networks (CNNs), which utilize either supervised or unsupervised training procedures [40]. The MLP network provides pattern recognition, optimization aids, process identification, and controls based on training in a single direction to enable universal pattern classifications. RNNs are networks with a closed loop, capable of memorizing and storing information, such as Boltzmann constants and Hopfield networks [41]. CNNs are a series of dynamic systems with local connections characterized by their topology. They have been used in image and video processing, biological system modeling, processing complex brain functions, pattern recognition, and sophisticated signal processing. The more complex forms include Kohonen, RBF, LVQ, counter-propagation, and ADALINE networks.

AI modeling can significantly reduce preclinical work. The prediction of the toxicity of any drug molecule is vital to avoid toxic effects, as predicted by LimTox, pkCSM, admetSAR, and Toxtree, which are available to help reduce the cost [42]. Advanced AI-based approaches look for compounds' similarities or project the compound's toxicity based on input features. The Tox21 Data Challenge organized by the National Institutes of Health, Environmental Protection Agency, and US Food and Drug Administration (FDA) was an initiative to evaluate several computational techniques to forecast the toxicity of thousands of environmental compounds and drugs; an ML algorithm named DeepTox outperformed all methods by identifying static and dynamic features within the chemical descriptors of the molecules, such as molecular weight and Van der Waals volume. It could efficiently predict the toxicity of a molecule based on predefined 2,500 toxicophore features [43].

Drug–protein interactions can also predict the chances of poly-pharmacology, which is the tendency of a drug molecule to interact with multiple receptors producing off-target adverse effects [44].

Traditional drug discovery projects relying on in vitro high-throughput screening (HTS) involve large investments and sophisticated experimental setups, affordable only to big biopharmaceutical companies. In this scenario, the application of efficient state-of-the-art computational methods and modern AI-based algorithms for rapid screening of repurposable chemical space, approved drugs, and natural products with proven pharmacokinetic profiles to identify the initial leads is a powerful option to save resources and time. Structure-based drug repurposing is popular in silico repurposing approach [45].

Developing novel inhibitors against discoidin domain receptor-1 (DDR1) within 46 days and cyclin-dependent kinase-20 (CDK20) as a potential anti-lung-cancer drug within 30 days through AI-driven models is a remarkable proof of 'intelligent' drug discovery [46,47]. AI-driven repurposing is many folds faster than the traditional method. The lock and key analogy (Figure 6.3) demonstrates the main challenges for AI in drug reinvention [48]. In contrast to the conventional method of target search, AI-driven methods enable screening of a larger number of locks (targets) and enable testing of available keys (small molecules) through virtual screening in a shorter period. It enables discovery, development, optimization, reinventing, and in silico testing of the exact key for target molecules.

Lock and key analogy showing the five main challenges for AI in drug discovery

LOCK AND KEY ANALOGY

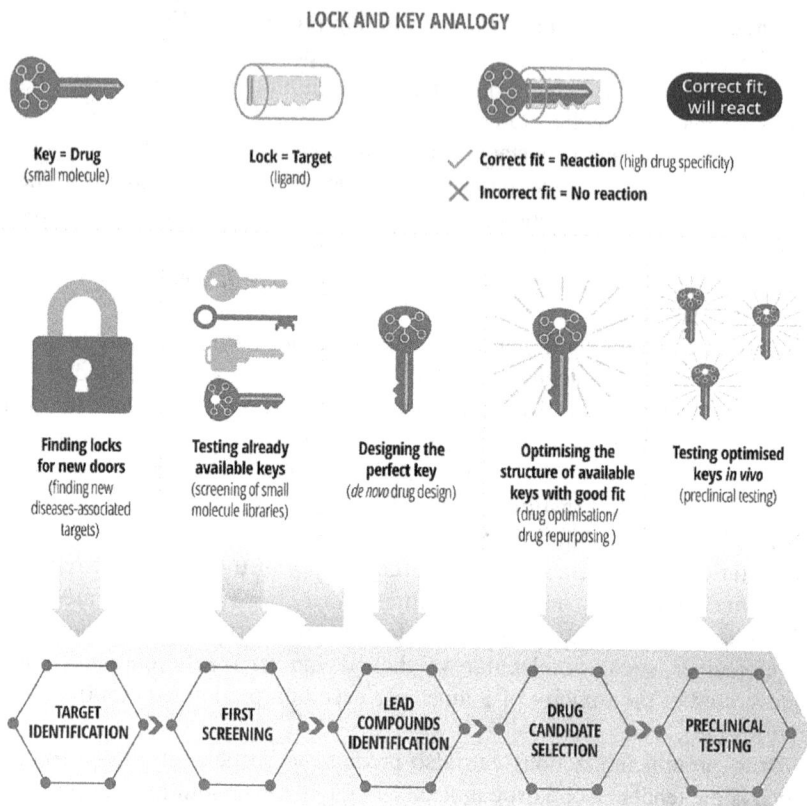

FIGURE 6.3 Lock and key analogy of challenges for AI in drug discovery [48].

While a protein may have been identified for a specific pharmacological response, much of the landscape of protein structure as domains remains unexplored; discovering a new key will expand the utility of an approved therapeutic protein (Figure 6.3).

AI-directed methods can further automate lead optimization, improve drug safety, design molecules with specific properties, and scrutinize structural databases to design poly-pharmacological and multi-target agents.

6.6 STRUCTURE PREDICTION

Finding domains that can bind starts with a detailed structural analysis. Experimental methods for protein structure identification include X-ray crystallography, nuclear magnetic resonance, cryo-electron microscopy, circular dichroism spectroscopy, etc. [49,50]. However, the testing variability of these methods depends on the quality of samples and precision of equipment, and the results can be compared with the data reported in UniProt and RCSB Protein Databank (PDB); currently, the PDB has approximately 174,825 experimentally derived structures available for comparison [51].

With major advancements in ML and AI, template-free protein structure prediction methods have also increased the accuracy and reliability of structure prediction methods. Template-free AI models are trained on the sequence and structural data from openly available databases, i.e., UniProt, RCSB PDB, Uniclust [52], BFD [53], MGnify [54], etc. Highly accurate protein structure prediction tools independent of templates include AlphaFold2 [55], trTosetta [56,57], Robetta [58], RoseTTA Fold [59], ESMFold [60], and OmegaFold [61]. Each algorithm uses a different AI model to predict protein structures from amino acid sequences. For example, AlphaFold2 uses a deep neural network-based approach with over 200 million protein structures openly available in the AlphaFold2 database [62]. trRosetta uses transfer learning with pre-trained deep neural networks; the Robetta server combines ab initio and homology-based methods with ML algorithms.

In contrast, RoseTTA Fold combines the strengths of Rosetta and deep neural networks. In addition, ESMFold uses energy-based statistical mechanical and language models, and OmegaFold integrates a protein language model with an end-to-end DL framework. These variations allow an orthogonal approach to predict the structure, providing greater reliability of the results. As a result, AI-based structure prediction tools have accelerated the process of therapeutic protein reinvention.

For some proteins, the structure can be predicted through template-based homology modeling, protein threading, and ab initio methods with the assistance of computational tools, i.e., I-TESSER [63,64], SWISS-MODEL [65], MODELLER [66], etc. Despite the significant differences in the specific procedures used by these prediction methods, the underlying steps are similar, including template selection, structure reconstruction, refinement, and analysis [67].

AI-driven retrosynthetic routes [68], phenotypic data or disease data, and molecule network-based algorithms without much structural data are used to design structures that can bind to the interface of targets while controlling their solubility [69,70] and benchmarking antibody discovery through AlphaFold2-enabled molecular docking and simulations [71]. One of the most remarkable events of AI-driven drug discovery was the application of AlphaFold2, PandaOmics [72] in discovering a small molecule target against CDK20 with a binding affinity of $9.2 \pm 0.5 \mu M$ ($n=3$), designed and tested in only 30 days [47].

6.7 TARGET IDENTIFICATION

In the on-target strategy, a new indication of the drug acting through the originally known target is explored since the mechanism of action is expected to retain the same therapeutic effects. In the off-target strategy, new drug uses are identified acting through an unanticipated target; in this case, the mechanism of action is not apparent. Docking and fingerprinting are standard methods.

The use of AI tools in drug–target identification has dramatically improved the efficiency of drug reinventions by enabling the concurrent screening of active compounds and predicting potential drug targets with greater accuracy. AI-based tools have revolutionized how pharmaceutical companies approach discoveries, significantly reducing the time, cost, error, and bias in finding new disease treatments.

HTS has long been a popular method in drug–target identification. Based on hit and trial, chemical compounds are screened against potential targets to identify compounds with desirable pharmacological properties. More precise target-based screening methods comprise identifying and developing molecules against specific targets, followed by phenotypic screening by screening compounds against cells or tissues. These discovery techniques have previously overcome the needle-in-the-haystack probabilities of such searches.

Under development are many new AI tools for screening active compounds in the search for hit compounds and enhancing the efficiency of the development process [73].

AtomNet is a CNN-based tool that applies the concepts of feature locality and hierarchical composition extracted through protein sequence, structure, and function to model bioactivity and chemical interactions of potential drug targets [74]. AtomNet's parent AtomWise has recently enabled the rapid discovery of drugs against 27 disease targets. DeepDTA is also a deep-learning-based model that uses only sequence information of targets and drugs to predict DTI binding affinities and potential small molecules as drug candidates from given biological data [75].

A commercially available natural compounds database and search engine that operates using ML, MolPort, when used with quantitative–structure–activity relationship (QSAR), analyze the chemical structure and predicts the biological activity of potential targets in the early stages of drug discovery [76].

Pathway analysis also enables the identification of potential targets. Some crucial biological pathways are available on the Kegg Pathway database [77], which provides insight into a disease mechanism. TargetNet [78] uses this pathway data and protein interaction profiles to predict potential drug targets against a specific disease.

DeepDock is the most recent AI-driven virtual screening platform with a vast library of small molecules. For example, DeepDock virtual screen results were used to identify 15% active molecules that led to the discovery of novel compounds against the Mpro protease of SARS-CoV2 [79].

6.8 MOLECULAR DOCKING

Identifying structure, functional regions, interaction profiles, and immune system responses are crucial for the success of a therapeutic protein reaching the patients. Therefore, researchers have redirected their attention from conventional drug discovery methods to computational techniques to find new and effective therapeutic agents quickly.

Proteins interact with their receptors to initiate therapeutic effects and manipulate disease mechanisms. For years, fluorescence-based assays, isothermal titration calorimetry, surface plasmon resonance, NMR, and other methods have been used to study the binding patterns and thermodynamic effects of DTIs. While highly relevant for characterizing interactions, they are time-consuming, expensive, and resource-intensive. Using computational tools in molecular docking has expedited the drug discovery process exponentially, enabling repeated testing with the complexities of the classical method.

Structure-based drug discovery and ligand-based drug discovery both involve the identification of non-covalent interactions using molecular docking in the prediction of novel properties of therapeutic compounds following the lock-and-key hypothesis and induced-fit model [80,81]. In addition, both rely on molecular docking to predict the binding affinity and specificity of small molecules and their targets.

Advancements in computational techniques have led to more precise identification and optimization of binding mode, binding affinity, binding pocket, and solvation effects on DTIs.

Computer-based tools such as AutoDock Vina [82,83], LigandFit [84], UCSF DOCK [85], and GOLD [86] are widely used.

Higher binding affinity scores from an in-silico docking analysis of mAbs against Alpha and Delta strains of SARS-CoV spike protein suggested that tixagevimab, regdanvimab, and cilgavimab can neutralize most Alpha strains efficiently and bamlanivimab, tixagevimab, and sotrovimab can be effective in suppressing the Delta strain [87]. Venetoclax [88], for treating chronic lymphocytic leukemia, was designed to target the overexpressed BCL-2 protein in cancer cells by binding to its hydrophobic groove. Its development involved optimizing the binding interactions between the drug and BCL-2 through in-silico docking studies, highlighting the importance of docking in drug design.

Computational techniques have enabled the targeted discovery of drugs through detailed interaction studies instead of blind docking. However, the precision of these interactions is highly dependent on the pose generation algorithms, binding pocket identification, and scoring functions. In addition, therapeutic targets, such as proteins and ligands, have a large conformational degree of freedom, resulting in extensive data to analyze.

Docking programs sample works through variable methods by treating ligands as flexible or proteins as flexible or/and, in some cases, both as flexible.

GOLD uses a genetic algorithm, and Autodock Vina uses a grid-based energy approach with a genetic algorithm.

ICM [89] uses multiple stochastic runs.

GLIDE SP [90] uses several sampling and scoring methods.

DeepBSP, an ML-based sampling and evaluation tool, is very useful in generating and ranking profiles close to their respective native structures as an ML model-based pose sampling and evaluation [91].

Identification of the correct view is crucial for higher binding affinity and lower steric hindrance, which can be efficiently achieved through precise AI-based tools. Structure prediction tools such as AlphaFold2 and trRosetta can be integrated with other ML-based approaches to identify and optimize potential poses. One such instance is identifying transition states between the active and inactive conformations of G-protein coupled receptors using multiple ML approaches [92].

The effectiveness of interaction between the dynamic views and their binding partners can be weighted through scoring systems. Scoring functions are categorized into force-field-based, knowledge-based, and empirical scoring functions.

Force-field-based scoring functions utilize molecular mechanics to evaluate complex energetic affinities based on their interactions, i.e., weak Van der Waals, electrostatic forces, bond stretching, bending, and torsional angles [93].

Knowledge-based scoring functions include statistical analysis of distance-dependent atom-pair potentials of protein–ligand or protein–protein complexes generated directly from experimental structures [94,95]. Empirical scoring functions, e.g., LUDI [96], ID-Score [97], and GlideScore [90], are based on empirical data. They correlate binding free energies to weak Van der Waals energy, electrostatic energy, desolvation, entropy, enthalpy, H-bonding, rotational and translational degrees of freedom, polar and lipophilic effects, and hydrophobicity in the form of simple equations to reproduce experimental affinity data.

These scores are used in combinations for better optimization, i.e., DockThor programs DockTScore [94,98] and blends empirical and force-field-based scoring methods, SMoG2016 [99] fuses empirical and knowledge-based scoring methods, and GalaxyDock BP2 Score [100] uses all three: force-field-based, knowledge-based, and empirical scoring methods [94].

The recent integration of physics-based terms and ML in DockTScore has further enhanced binding energy prediction and conformation ranking [101].

GNINA docking software, based on an ensemble of CNNs as a scoring function for scoring the sample view, has outperformed AutoDock Vina [102], once again proving that the paradigm shift from conventional methods to AI-based methods has significantly increased the impartial interpretations of scientific evidence leading to the discovery of targets.

6.8.1 Limitations

Despite its many advantages, the application of AI faces data challenges, such as the data's scale, growth, diversity, and uncertainty. The data sets available for drug development in pharmaceutical companies can involve millions of compounds, and traditional ML tools might be unable to deal with these data types. The recent natural language-based AI tools, such as the GPT4, are anticipated to resolve some of these issues.

While the QSAR-based computational model can quickly predict large numbers of compounds or simple physicochemical parameters, such as log P or log D, predicting biological properties remains challenging. These limitations will be reduced when larger training sets, experimental validation, and more data error training are added in the future.

AI-based data analysis significantly reduces the burden of research and testing in the early discovery phase, as it can handle a large volume of data for profiling molecules. However, it does stand to replace efficacy testing in patients [103] due to the safety issues that form the basis of the regulatory requirements. However, it does significantly decrease the work leading to clinical efficacy testing.

6.8.1.1 Structure Modifications

Optimization of the safety and efficacy of drug candidates is a critical step in the drug development process. One approach to optimizing a protein-based drug is to truncate it to enhance its selectivity, potency, and PK–PDc properties. Truncation of proteins has been widely used to develop more effective therapeutics and has proven to be a successful strategy in improving bioavailability. Additionally, the optimization of drugs can be combined with reinventing drug strategies to identify new therapeutic uses for existing drugs.

Recently, anti-rheumatoid arthritis effects of native Staphylococcal protein (SpA), recombinant full-length SpA, and a truncated form of SpA were used in a comparative study along with Enbrel (commercial drug) to test reduction in several inflammatory cytokines (IL-8, IL-1β, TNF-α, and IL-6). The truncated SpA had a higher efficacy even when compared to Enbrel. Another study suggested that exogenous truncated inhibitor K562 protein (tIK) has the potential to act as a new therapeutic in patients with Enbrel resistance since their modes of action are contrary to each other [104]. Furthermore, in vivo and silico analyses suggest that the truncated protein resulted in the exposure of the IgG-binding domain, which led to effective binding through an increased radius of gyration [105]. Similar studies have been conducted previously as well.

The N-terminal truncated recombinant form of fibroblast growth factor 21 (FGF 21: amino acids 30–210) demonstrated improved stability and PK in obsess-mouse models. In more than one species of mouse, recombinant FGF21 (Fc-FGF21(RG)) administered once per week produced a similar or higher response than human FGF21 (hrFGF21) administered daily [106,107]. Furthermore, interleukin-2 (IL-2), a cytokine that stimulates the activation of immune cells, has been optimized by truncating the N-terminal region containing a binding site for IL-2 receptor alpha to produce NKTR-214. NKTR-214 has enhanced selectivity and potency, increasing efficacy against tumor cells [108].

6.9   DRUG CONJUGATES

Chemotherapy damages healthy cells that can be protected by using antibody–drug conjugates (ADCs) that direct chemotherapy towards only cancer cells, making it safer [109–111]. The ADCs deliver chemotherapy when a linker connected to a monoclonal antibody binds to a particular target expressed in cancer cells. After binding to the target (cancer protein or receptor), the ADC releases a cytotoxic drug into the cancer cell. "Fully human" mAbs engineered to carry human antibody genes are an ideal delivery platform for ADCs. They are highly targeted and cell specific, have an extended circulating half-life, and offer minimal immunogenicity. The chemical "linkers" that combine the antibodies and cytotoxic drugs are highly stable to prevent cleaving (splitting) before the ADC enters the tumor. Anticancer drugs (or "payloads") penetrate the tumor and cause cell death by damaging the DNA of cancer cells or preventing new cancer cells from forming and spreading (Figure 6.4).

The FDA has approved 14 ADCs, while the EMA has approved 8; about 300 are under development [112], mostly for oncological and hematological indications. However, these applications can be expanded to other important disease areas [113]. For example, the payloads for oncology ADCs (oADC) can be derived from natural sources, including the microtubulin inhibitors monomethyl auristatin A MMAE [114], monomethyl auristatin F MMAF [115], mertansine, DNA binder calicheamicin [116], topoisomerase 1 inhibitor SN-38 [117], and exatecan [118].

Chemical motif-defined linkers include disulfides, hydrazones, peptides (cleavable), or thioethers (non-cleavable). Cleavable and non-cleavable linkers have proven

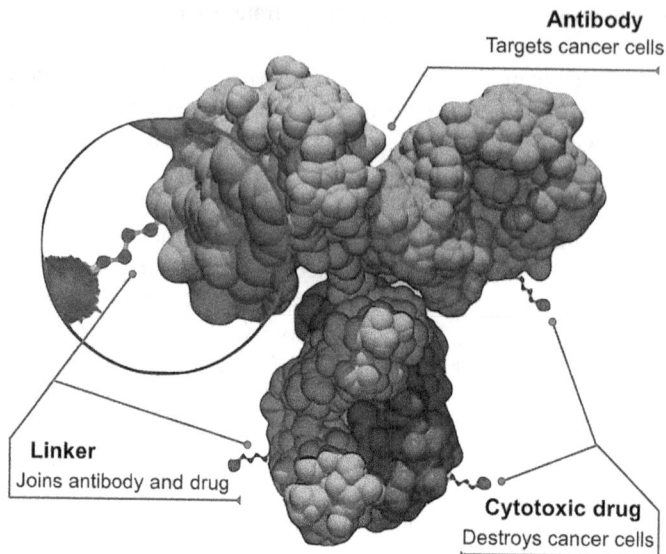

FIGURE 6.4 Drug-antibody conjugate design. By Bioconjugator—Own work, CC BY-SA 4.0, https://commons.wikimedia.org/w/index.php?curid=58772304.

safe in preclinical and clinical trials. The anti-microtubule agent monomethyl auristatin E, or Monomethyl auristatin E (MMAE), a synthetic antineoplastic agent, is delivered to human-specific CD30-positive malignant cells by the enzyme-sensitive cleavable linker in the drug compound brentuximab vedotin. By preventing the polymerization of tubulin, MMAE prevents cell division. MMAE cannot be utilized as a single-agent chemotherapeutic medication due to its severe toxicity. However, the stability of MMAE attached to an anti-CD30 monoclonal antibody is unaffected by extracellular fluid. Trastuzumab emtansine combines the microtubule-formation inhibitor mertansine (DM-1) and antibody trastuzumab, which uses a non-cleavable stable linker [119].

Due to the availability of newer and more robust linkers, the function of the chemical bond has changed. The linker's cleavable or non-cleavable nature determines the cytotoxic medication's characteristics. A non-cleavable linker, for instance, retains the medicine inside the cell. As a result, the entire antibody complex—including the linker and the cytotoxic (anti-cancer) agent—enters the cancer cell that is being targeted, where the antibody is broken down into an amino acid. The resulting complex, which consists of an amino acid, a linker, and a cytotoxic agent, is regarded as an active medication. On the other hand, cleavable linkers are dissociated by cancer cell enzymes. The cytotoxic payload can then leave the targeted cell and destroy nearby cells through a process known as "bystander killing" [120].

AOCs, or antibody-oligonucleotide conjugates, comprise two essential classes of macromolecules: mAbs and oligonucleotides. With AOC, various applications, such as imaging, detection, and targeted therapeutics, have profited from the union of the diverse functional modes of oligonucleotides with the potent targeting properties of mAbs. The fundamental obstacles to effective ON therapies are cell internalization and absorption. ADCs can be used to get around problems with administering and internalizing ON therapies. The bioconjugation process has been used to obtain several such conjugates.

The utility of ADCs and AOCs is limited to solid tumors because of the larger physical size (150 kDa) since the antibody size cannot be modified [121]. Therefore, nanobody–ON conjugates are intensively used to exploit the small nanobody size to reduce imaging displacement [122].

6.9.1 RADIOIMMUNOCONJUGATES (RIC)

Radiation is an effective therapy for many tumor types. However, external beam radiation therapy is associated with many nonspecific side effects. Modern radiation techniques such as intensity-modulated and proton beam therapy have increased precision, delivered higher radiation dosages, and reduced toxicities to the surrounding tissues [123] (Figure 6.5).

Radioimmunotherapy (RIT) has been explored as a cancer therapeutic for many decades [124]. RIT utilizes antibodies directed at an antigen expressed on the tumor cell surface to deliver cytotoxic radionuclides that emit α or β particles to the tumor sites. After the radioimmunoconjugates (RICs) bind to the surface antigen on the tumor cells, the α or β particles emitted by the radionuclides induce DNA damage and trigger tumor cell apoptosis [125]. RICs have been viewed mainly as a radiation delivery system to treat metastatic cancer unsuitable for an external beam approach. RICs aim to increase the radiation specificity and allow for the delivery of higher radiation dosages with fewer toxicities. However, the current understanding of tumor immunology suggests that RICs may be more than just a radiation delivery system and present a fertile field for reinventing therapeutic proteins.

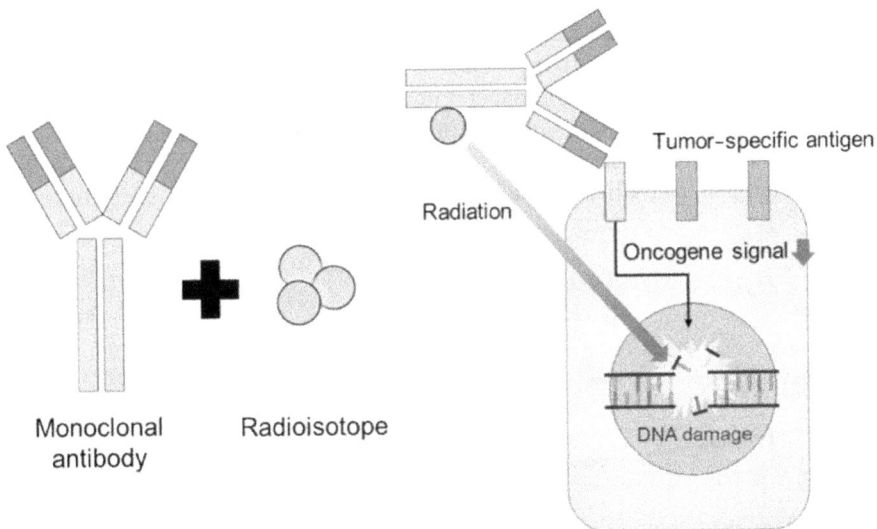

FIGURE 6.5 Design and function of radioimmune therapies [127].

Because of their high cytotoxic potential, RICs emitting α- or β-particles can be used for targeted cancer therapy. Cancer treatment using RICs requires careful consideration of the choice of radionuclides and their dosage. β-emitters have a deeper penetration range and a lower linear energy transfer (LET) than α-emitters, whereas α-particles can release high energy at a relatively shorter distance. However, while α-particles are more efficient in tumor cell eradication without causing much collateral damage, β-particles are currently most commonly used in radioimmunotherapy. Many β-emitters, such as 131I and 90Y, are commercially available and have established techniques for conjugating them to antibodies. For example, 90Y-ibritumomab tiuxetan and 131I-tositumomab are US FDA-approved RICs targeting CD20 for treating B-cell non-Hodgkin lymphoma [126]. α-Emitters, on the other hand, are not widely commercially available, techniques for conjugating them to antibodies are not well-established, and PK and dosimetry of α-emitters need further investigation for clinical applications. Large-scale production of radionuclides, especially α-emitters, for clinical applications, requires a significant investment.

RICs consist of a targeting antibody conjugated to a radionuclide chelator and indirectly labeled with a radionuclide. The two most commonly used chelators are trans-(S, S)-cyclohexane-diethylenetriamine pentaacetate (CHX-A″-DTPA) and dodecane tetraacetate (DOTA) [127]. In addition, various radionuclides have been used, including ^{131}I, ^{111}In, ^{90}Y, ^{225}Ac, and ^{177}Lu. RICs combine radiation's cytotoxicity with antibodies' specificity to provide powerful antitumor effects to patients with metastatic cancer.

Conventional antibodies directed at intact proteins enable targeting antigens expressed on the surface of tumor cells (Figure 6.6). If TCR-like antibodies directed at antigen peptides/MHC complexes are used instead, they are also suitable for targeting intracellular antigens. As long as a tumor type is radiosensitive, a wide range of radioisotopes may be chelated to the antibodies, including those emitting α or β emitting particles. An ideal radioisotope would have a short half-life, appropriate penetration range, and high LET. In addition to their cytotoxic potential, RICs may be a comprehensive immunotherapeutic agent not limited by the obstacles currently hindering the success of modern cancer immunotherapy. Unlike antibody–drug conjugates, RICs do not require cellular internalization to induce tumor cell kill because of their relatively larger decay sphere of penetration. They circumvent the obstacles related to antigen internalization and uptake of the drug due to lysosomal dysfunction

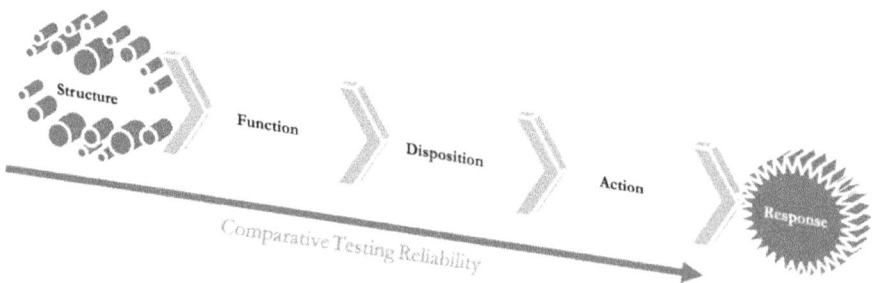

FIGURE 6.6 The ladder of objectivity from the highest to the lowest.

and drug efflux pumps. In this section, we will discuss the wide range of effects of RICs and how they may be harnessed for effective and more specific cancer therapy.

Only a few active and recruiting studies for non-hematologic solid tumors are registered with Clinicaltrials.gov. The FDA-approved products include Ibritumomab tiuxetan (Zevalin), a monoclonal antibody anti-CD20 conjugated to a molecule that chelates Yttrium-90; Iodine (^{131}I) tositumomab (Bexxar) that links a molecule containing Iodine-131 to an anti-CD20 monoclonal antibody, and now withdrawn; and Lutetium (^{177}Lu) lilotomab satetraxetan (Betalutin), a combination of lutetium-177 and an anti-CD37 monoclonal antibody.

6.10 REGULATORY PERSPECTIVE

The success of reinventing therapeutic proteins depends significantly on how the regulatory agencies evaluate these products. Sometimes, these are a new class of drugs for which the agencies may need a guideline. In other cases, the agencies may be highly conservative, a mindset that is the responsibility of the developers to change by offering detailed educational discussion in the filing.

The critical reasons for the failure of new drug discoveries include inadequate efficacy or safety, lack of target validation, or inability to meet regulatory requirements. Although computational Drug Design has significantly reduced the chances of riskier drugs entering clinical trials and conserves resources, this should be emphasized in the regulatory filing with justification.

The FDA is leading the perspective of introducing new techniques in structure prediction, target identification, and interaction profiling to revolutionize drug development, setting the industry's standard for precision and efficiency [128]. Recently, these efforts have identified the source of acute kidney injury or hepatic injury from using remdesivir in COVID-19 treatment using a target-prediction software followed by QSAR and structure similarity analysis to identify an association between the structure of metabolites and renal-hepatic toxicity [129].

Using AI, the FDA has developed models to classify and clinically monitor organ systems more prone to toxicity [130] and is currently developing natural language processing algorithms to identify molecular targets associated with pediatric cancer through peer-reviewed literature. In addition, the FDA is conducting research within its Division of Applied Regulatory Science (DARS) program [131].

The DARS is also researching the efficacy of non-clinical methods for anticipating immunogenicity risk. This entails analyzing in vitro assays and cell types, developing in vivo models, and selecting proper controls.

The DARS has also experimented with cutting-edge non-clinical models to forecast cytokine release syndrome, a potentially fatal side effect linked to biological products [132,133], and showed that non-clinical models could effectively demonstrate this adverse event. Furthermore, checkpoint inhibitor oncology therapies for which adverse events cannot be predicted using computational, in vitro, or conventional non-clinical methods can be studied further after successfully demonstrating immune-mediated activation in a non-clinical model [134].

DARS places much emphasis on using molecular target information to anticipate safety issues. Knowing a drug's molecular targets enables early detection of its effects and potential safety issues for new molecules. Still, the exact modeling can also be applied in a comparator mode to study biosimilar candidates. For instance, DARS created several computational techniques, such as ML, to forecast a drug's negative effects based on the biological receptors that the drug, or other medications with a similar structure, are known to target [135,136]. These computational methodologies are proving promising in predicting adverse events.

A database for secondary pharmacology activity provided by the industry as part of their application for an investigational new drug is also being built and analyzed by DARS. A drug developer typically performs in vitro target binding and functional assays for 80–100 biological receptors to ascertain potential on-target and off-target effects. However, the targets chosen for the assays and submission format are not currently standardized across the industry. Therefore, data from these assays have been manually extracted and curated into a database to allow easier access and analysis of these study results. Additionally, DARS is engaging in a public–private partnership with the Pistoia Alliance [137] to choose the most effective procedures for submitting these studies to regulatory bodies in the future.

Other issues that the DARS is resolving include using a state-of-the-art alternative to experimental testing to qualify a drug impurity for mutagenic potential [138]. This can significantly help when a biosimilar candidate shows an unmatched impurity. The FDA has suggested using flow imaging microscopy (FIM) to record and analyze images using CNNs or ConvNets [139]. In addition, the FDA has suggested ParticleSentry AI software [140] to analyze the data to enable protein aggregation profiling.

6.10.1 REGULATORY SUBMISSION

Theoretically, the regulatory agencies will treat a reinvented product as a new drug application, and the developer must submit all information required for a new molecule. However, regulatory agencies also allow the submission of information in the public domain, such as the registration dossiers of the selected therapeutic protein from the FDA [141] or EMA [142] portals or the EPARs in the EMA. This leads to a creative approach, "351(a) modified" [143], a term crafted by the authors to significantly reduce the cost and time to approval. Furthermore, even when a therapeutic protein is combined with another drug or a radioactive source, the studies specific to the safety of the therapeutic protein are significantly reduced, making reinventing therapeutic proteins the most efficient and creative path to bringing in new affordable treatment modalities.

6.10.2 NONCLINICAL TESTING

Figure 6.6 shows a dependency model leading from receptor binding to patient efficacy. As we move further down the slope, the testing becomes more subjective and less objective, making it a sound argument why a test with higher sensitivity should be reconfirmed with a lesser sensitivity test. Receptor binding remains the most robust and convincing test to demonstrate the safety and efficacy of therapeutic proteins. The receptor binding need not demonstrate a known PD marker, and the marker must correlate with the clinical response. This relationship forms the basis of the thesis that receptor binding alone can be used to substitute clinical efficacy testing; there is no need for the developers to investigate and find a PD marker either.

The drug approval dossiers and published literature disclose study designs employed in establishing safety and efficacy data of new products; these study models should be replicated for the reinvented product to avoid regulatory approval delays. Further modeling and simulation can provide the dose–response relationships, sensitive dose ranges, population sensitivity, and variability in PD biomarker responses [144–148].

6.10.3 PHARMACOKINETICS–PHARMACODYNAMICS

Another consideration that can significantly improve the PK/PD data is the inclusion criteria of the test subjects; choosing a narrow characteristic population regarding age, gender, BMI, ethnicity, and pharmacogenomics to antibody responses can significantly reduce the study size and add substantial validity to the data [149].

The PK studies can further support the PD marker utility by extending the data analysis to demonstrate how fast and how much of the parenterally administered drug is leaving the central compartment, thus reaching out to receptor sites; this analysis will demonstrate a similarity in the onset of action. In addition, this property can be compared by adding a pharmacokinetic parameter, the rate of change of distribution volume as a function of time [150], applied in several clinical efficacy comparisons based on clearance and tissue binding [151].

Binding affinities to target antigens can significantly influence the PK of mAbs, requiring measurements of affinity or equilibrium dissociation constant (Kd), association rate constant (kon), and dissociation rate constant (koff). There is an optimal binding affinity beyond which the distribution of the mAb to target tissue may be impaired [152,153]. This affinity is readily established by the characterization of binding to FcRn; as this is a pH-dependent interaction, binding affinity should be measured at pH 6.0 (where FcRn binds mAb in the acidic pH of the endosome) and pH 7.4 (physiological pH where FcRn releases mAb at the cell surface). High binding to FcRn at pH 6.0 and low binding at pH 7.4 is essential for low clearance of mAbs [154,155]. Several studies have investigated the correlation between FcRn binding affinity and the half-life of mAbs, and the contribution of FcRn to prolonging the half-lives of mAbs is well recognized [156]. Since the PK of mAbs depends on PD [157,158], the PK profile projects the PD properties, making it reflective of the PD.

Specifically, pharmacokinetic models should represent physiological variables, and levels of unbound drugs in body fluids should receive greater emphasis [159]. Furthermore, the degree of plasma protein binding, in turn, influences the distribution, action, metabolism, and renal excretion, and most importantly, the distribution triggers that response [160].

14C-labeled reworked product testing is an excellent tool to demonstrate changes in the disposition profile, and the FDA highly recommends such studies [161].

For reducing side effects, dose changes can be helpful. These changes are best justified based on the characterization of ADMET (Absorption, Distribution, Metabolism, Excretion, and toxicity). An aphorism written by Nicholas Holford and Lewis Sheiner in 1982, "Pharmacokinetics is what the body does to the drug; PD is what the drug does to the body" [162], fully describes these terms. PK is the movement of the drug across the membranes of cells, and PD is its interaction with potential biological targets. Collectively, they provide insight into desired therapeutic effects and, sometimes, undesired effects, i.e., toxicity and immunogenic responses. The administered substance goes through a cascade of events inside the body to be efficacious.

Molecular interactions data and the PK/PD profiles can be used along with AI models to automate the pharmacovigilance process, pre-clinical and post-clinical surveillance, design efficient clinical trials, suggest the optimal route of administration, and facilitate the selection of highly effective dose regimens.

Discovering and identifying specific binding site poses and affinities results in lower off-target binding, toxicity, and immunogenicity. Preclinical PK/PD analysis, mapping dose–response relationships of exposure, and biological effects in the plasma and target tissue can significantly enhance drug discovery. The effective concentration of the drug in the plasma and the maximum effect is plotted against time, using single or multi-compartment models to characterize PK/PD effects.

PK modeling has proven to be significant in predicting plasma exposure of therapeutics, i.e., if a single 10 mg/kg dose response is known in a mouse model, modeling could help predict the effects of twice-a-day 30 mg/kg dose to hypothesize and optimize a dosing regimen. The PK/PD properties of therapeutic mAbs differ from that of small molecules; hence the concentration of free ligands can be an established marker of their efficacy. Clinically tested effects of galcanezumab dose (120 and 240 mg), validated through PK modeling, indicated a steady decrease in the concentration of free ligands resulting in the development of efficacious dose regimens [163]. A PK and target engagement (molecular interaction) study of anti-interferon-γ-induced protein 10 (IP-10) mAb was characterized, which concluded optimal dose strategy and scheduling of drug administration, i.e., approximately eight subcutaneously delivered dose intervals were required weekly in this case to reach steady state [164].

6.10.4 FUNCTION TESTING

Specialized cell-based bioassays or potency assays, including ELISA, binding assays, competitive assays, cell signaling, ligand binding, proliferation, and proliferation suppression, are essential in ascertaining the mechanism of action and similarity with the parent molecule. On the other hand, functional tests related to the possible MOA, such as apoptosis, complement-dependent cytotoxicity, antibody-dependent cellular phagocytosis, and antibody-dependent cellular cytotoxicity, among others, are necessary but not essential, especially when it is not relevant. For instance, functional tests (ADCC, ADCP, and CDC) are unnecessary for a product that predominantly targets a soluble antigen [165–169].

Thus, comparable bioassay results should be sufficient when PD markers are unavailable, such as for mAbs. Therefore, a complete bioassay toolbox is a crucial enabler for applying the proposed clinical development paradigm. The toolbox requires multiple assays, ideally cell-based, to cover all relevant functions of a molecule with accurate and precise quantitative readouts and agreement with the regulators on the bioassay designs, including their validation [170,171]. For example, comparable binding affinities to TNF-α, Clq complement, and a complete panel of Fc-receptors for etanercept have proven sufficient to establish biosimilarity since this binding is the primary mechanism of action of etanercept [172].

For a product with multiple biological activities, a set of relevant functional assays designed to evaluate the range of activities of the product can be tested. For example, specific proteins possess multiple functional domains that express enzymatic and receptor-binding activities. Potency is the measure of biological activity. When immunochemical properties are part of the activity attributed to the product (for example, antibodies or antibody-based products), analytical tests to characterize these properties are readily available.

6.10.5   IMMUNOGENIC RESPONSE

Proteins are immunogenic and capable of producing neutralizing antibodies (NAbs) that bind to drug products and may diminish or eliminate the associated biological activity; these are unintended and undesirable outcomes. Standard immunoassays can detect drug-specific antibodies but cannot distinguish NAbs. Therefore, cell-based assays are often preferred because they closely mimic the mechanism by which NAbs and drug products interact in vivo. However, each cell-based NAb assay is unique and based on several factors, such as the drug product, study population, and development phase (preclinical or clinical). In addition, the type of NAb assay (direct or indirect) depends on the drug's mechanism of action. Generally, the appearance of NAbs is not a pivotal issue if their presence does not alter the disposition profile, such as in the case of insulin [173]. Reinvented products should be compared with the original product to ensure that the changes made, either in structure or combination compositions, do not alter the NAb level or immunogenicity.

6.11   CONCLUSIONS

The higher attrition rate of new drug discovery from conventional methods leads to a wastage of resources and time after hefty preclinical and clinical testing [174]. As a result, the cost of new drug development has skyrocketed over the past decade into billions of dollars [175]. Compared to chemical drugs, therapeutic proteins present a remarkable opportunity to reinvent their use because of their mechanism of action—receptor binding—and vast structure that presents hundreds of possibilities for finding new uses of an approved therapeutic protein. Billions of dollars of markets are thus available without spending the billions and providing new therapies at a much lower cost when the approved therapeutic proteins are put into a reinvention cycle. This exercise was much more difficult until a decade ago when AI and ML systems entered the field of science. HTS enabled identifying potential targets using in silico approaches. As a result, the regulatory burden of the reinvented products is substantially less than a new molecule, and so are the risks of failure.

It is strongly urged that developers, both large and small, investigate this remarkable treasure of therapies available to explore at a highly affordable cost and bring therapies for thousands of rare and complex diseases.

REFERENCES

1. Raju, T.N. The Nobel Chronicles. 1988: James Whyte Black, (b 1924), Gertrude Elion (1918-99), and George H Hitchings (1905-98). *Lancet* 2000, 355, 1022.
2. Sean. (5 February 2023). The Process and Costs of Drug Development. FTLOScience. 2022. Available online: https://ftloscience.com/process-costs-drug-development/ (accessed on 30 March 2023).
3. Leenaars, C.H.C.; Kouwenaar, C.; Stafleu, F.R.; Bleich, A.; Ritskes-Hoitinga, M.; De Vries, R.B.M.; Meijboom, F.L.B. Animal to human translation: A systematic scoping review of reported concordance rates. *J. Transl. Med.* 2019, 17, 223. https://doi.org/10.1186/s12967-019-1976-2.
4. Papapetropoulos, A.; Szabo, C. Inventing new therapies without reinventing the wheel: The power of drug repurposing. *Br. J. Pharmacol.* 2018, 175, 165–167. https://doi.org/10.1111/bph.14081.
5. Pearce, R.M. Chance and the prepared mind. *Science* 1912, 35, 941–956. https://doi.org/10.1126/science.35.912.941.
6. Wermuth, C.G. Selective optimization of side activities: The SOSA approach. *Drug Discov. Today* 2006, 11, 160–164. https://doi.org/10.1016/s1359-6446(05)03686-x.
7. Prosdocimi, M.; Zuccato, C.; Cosenza, L.C.; Borgatti, M.; Lampronti, I.; Finotti, A.; Gambari, R. A rational approach to drug repositioning in β-thalassemia: Induction of fetal hemoglobin by established drugs. *Wellcome Open Res.* 2022, 7, 150. https://doi.org/10.12688/wellcomeopenres.17845.3.
8. Bomprezzi, R. Dimethyl fumarate in the treatment of relapsing-remitting multiple sclerosis: An overview. *Ther. Adv. Neurol. Disord.* 2015, 8, 20–30. https://doi.org/10.1177/1756285614564152.
9. Blair, H.A. Dimethyl fumarate: A review in moderate to severe plaque psoriasis. *Drugs* 2018, 78, 123–130. https://doi.org/10.1007/s40265-017-0854-6.
10. Santoro, M.G.; Carafoli, E. Remdesivir: From Ebola to COVID-19. *Biochem. Biophys. Res. Commun.* 2021, 538, 145–150. https://doi.org/10.1016/j.bbrc.2020.11.043.
11. Beck, B.R.; Shin, B.; Choi, Y.; Park, S.; Kang, K. Predicting commercially available antiviral drugs that may act on the novel coronavirus (SARS-CoV-2) through a drug-target interaction deep learning model. *Comput. Struct. Biotechnol. J.* 2020, 18, 784–790.
12. Gilvary, C.; Elkhader, J.; Madhukar, N.; Henchcliffe, C.; Goncalves, M.D.; Elemento, O. A machine learning and network framework to discover new indications for small molecules. *PLoS Comput. Biol.* 2020, 16, e1008098. https://doi.org/10.1371/journal.pcbi.1008098.
13. Peng, Y.; Wang, M.; Xu, Y.; Wu, Z.; Wang, J.; Zhang, C.; Liu, G.; Li, W.; Li, J.; Tang, Y. Drug repositioning by prediction of drug's anatomical therapeutic chemical code via network-based inference approaches. *Briefings Bioinform.* 2021, 22, 2058–2072. https://doi.org/10.1093/bib/bbaa027.
14. Cong, Y.; Shintani, M.; Imanari, F.; Osada, N.; Endo, T. A new approach to drug repurposing with two-stage prediction, machine learning, and unsupervised clustering of gene expression. *OMICS A J. Integr. Biol.* 2022, 26, 339–347. https://doi.org/10.1089/omi.2022.0026.
15. Russo, D.; Di Filippo, P.; Di Pillo, S.; Chiarelli, F.; Attanasi, M. New Indications of Biological Drugs in Allergic and Immunological Disorders: Beyond Asthma, Urticaria, and Atopic Dermatitis. *Biomedicines* **2023**, 11, 236.
16. Jackson, D.A.; Symons, R.H.; Berg, P. Biochemical method for inserting new genetic information into DNA of Simian Virus 40: Circular SV40 DNA molecules containing lambda phage genes and the galactose operon of Escherichia coli. *Proc. Natl. Acad. Sci. USA* 1972, 69, 2904–2909.

17. Berg, P.; Baltimore, D.; Boyer, H.W.; Cohen, S.N.; Davis, R.W.; Hogness, D.S.; Nathans, D.; Roblin, R.; Watson, J.D.; Weissman, S.; et al. Letter: Potential biohazards of recombinant DNA molecules. *Science* 1974, 185, 303.
18. Landgraf, W.; Sandow, J. Recombinant human insulins-clinical efficacy and safety in diabetes therapy. *Eur. Endocrinol.* 2016, 12, 12–17. https://doi.org/10.17925/EE.2016.12.01.12.
19. Usmani, S.S.; Bedi, G.; Samuel, J.S.; Singh, S.; Kalra, S.; Kumar, P.; Ahuja, A.A.; Sharma, M.; Gautam, A.; Raghava, G.P.S. THPdb: Database of FDA-approved peptide and protein therapeutics. *PLoS ONE* 2017, 12, e0181748. https://doi.org/10.1371/journal.pone.0181748.
20. Dimitrov, D.S. Therapeutic proteins. *Methods Mol. Biol.* 2012, 899, 1–26. https://doi.org/10.1007/978-1-61779-921-1_1.
21. Available online: https://www.biospace.com/article/biologics-market-size-to-hit-usd-719-94-billion-by-2030-/ (accessed on 30 March 2023).
22. FDA. Available online: https://www.fda.gov/media/107622/download (accessed on 30 March 2023).
23. Available online: https://www.ncbi.nlm.nih.gov/books/NBK562260/#:~:text=A%20peptide%20is%20a%20short,the%20building%20block%20of%20proteins (accessed on 30 March 2023).
24. Niazi, S.K. Molecular biosimilarity-an AI-driven paradigm shift. *Int. J. Mol. Sci.* 2022, 23, 10690. https://doi.org/10.3390/ijms231810690.
25. Zwanzig, R.; Szabo, A.; Bagchi, B. Levinthal's paradox. *Proc. Natl. Acad. Sci. USA* 1992, 89, 20–22. https://doi.org/10.1073/pnas.89.1.20.
26. Schmidt, T.; Bergner, A.; Schwede, T. Modelling three-dimensional protein structures for applications in drug design. *Drug Discov. Today* 2014, 19, 890–897. https://doi.org/10.1016/j.drudis.2013.10.027.
27. Tai, W.; He, L.; Zhang, X.; Pu, J.; Voronin, D.; Jiang, S.; Zhou, Y.; Du, L. Characterization of the receptor-binding domain (RBD) of 2019 novel coronavirus: Implication for development of RBD protein as a viral attachment inhibitor and vaccine. *Cell. Mol. Immunol.* 2020, 17, 613–620. https://doi.org/10.1038/s41423-020-0400-4.
28. Available online: https://www.cms.gov/monoclonal#:~:text=Monoclonal%20Antibodies%20to%20Treat%20Mild%2Dto%2DModerate%20COVID%2D19&text=On%20December%202023%2C%202022%2C%20the,with%20severe%20COVID%2D19%20illness (accessed on 30 March 2023).
29. Available online: https://www.ema.europa.eu/en/documents/product-information/avastin-epar-product-information_en.pdf (accessed on 30 March 2023).
30. Available online: https://www.ajmc.com/view/considerations-for-use-of-bevacizumab-vikg-in-wet-amd (accessed on 30 March 2023).
31. Hotzel, I.; Theil, F.-P.; Bernstein, L.J.; Prabhu, S.; Deng, R.; Quintana, L.; Lutman, J.; Sibia, R.; Chan, P.; Bumbaca, D.; et al. A strategy for risk mitigation of antibodies with fast clearance. *mAbs* 2012, 4, 753–760.
32. Sharma, T.W.; Patapoff, T.W.; Kabakoff, B.; Pai, S.; Hilario, E.; Zhang, B.; Li, C.; Borisov, O.; Kelley, R.F.; Chorny, I.; Zhou, J.Z.; et al. In silico selection of therapeutic antibodies for development: Viscosity, clearance, and chemical stability. *Proc. Natl. Acad. Sci. USA* 2014, 111, 18601–18606.
33. Lagassé, H.D.; Alexaki, A.; Simhadri, V.L.; Katagiri, N.H.; Jankowski, W.; Sauna, Z.E.; Kimchi-Sarfaty, C. Recent advances in (therapeutic protein) drug development. *F1000Research* 2017, 6, 113. https://doi.org/10.12688/f1000research.9970.1.
34. Cha, Y.; Erez, T.; Reynolds, I.J.; Kumar, D.; Ross, J.; Koytiger, G.; Kusko, R.; Zeskind, B.; Risso, S.; Kagan, E.; et al. Drug reinventing from the perspective of pharmaceutical companies. *Br. J. Pharmacol.* 2018, 175, 168–180.
35. Singh, T.U.; Parida, S.; Lingaraju, M.C.; Kesavan, M.; Kumar, D.; Singh, R.K. Drug reinventing approach to fight COVID-19. *Pharmacol. Rep.* 2020, 72, 1479–1508.

36. Santos, R.; Ursu, O.; Gaulton, A.; Bento, A.P.; Donadi, R.S.; Bologa, C.G.; Karlsson, A.; Al-Lazikani, B.; Hersey, A.; Oprea, T.I.; et al. A comprehensive map of molecular drug targets. *Nat. Rev. Drug Discov.* 2017, 16, 19–34. https://doi.org/10.1038/nrd.2016.230.

37. Available online: https://www.greyb.com/blog/biologics-patents-expiring-2022-2023-2024-2025-2026-2027/ (accessed on 30 March 2023).

38. Goode, R.; Chao, B. Biological patent thickets and delayed access to biosimilars, an American problem. *J. Law Biosci.* 2022, 9, lsac022. https://doi.org/10.1093/jlb/lsac022.

39. Beneke, F.; Mackenrodt, M.-O. Artificial intelligence and collusion. *IIC Int. Rev. Intellect. Prop. Compet. Law* 2019, 50, 109–134.

40. Bielecki, A.; Bielecki, A. Foundations of artificial neural networks. In *Models of Neurons and Perceptrons: Selected Problems and Challenges*, Janusz, K., Ed.; Springer International Publishing; Polish Academy of Sciences: Warsaw, Poland, 2019; pp. 15–28.

41. Da Silva, I.N. *Artificial Neural Networks*; Springer: Berlin/Heidelberg, 2017.

42. Yang, X.; Wang, Y.; Byrne, R.; Schneider, G.; Yang, S. Concepts of artificial intelligence for computer-assisted drug discovery. *Chem. Rev.* 2019, 119, 10520–10594. https://doi.org/10.1021/acs.chemrev.8b00728.

43. Mayr, A.; Klambauer, G.; Unterthiner, T.; Hochreiter, S. DeepTox: Toxicity prediction using deep learning. *Front. Environ. Sci.* 2016, 3, 80. https://doi.org/10.3389/fenvs.2015.00080.

44. Li, X.; Xu, Y.; Cui, H.; Huang, T.; Wang, D.; Lian, B.; Li, W.; Qin, G.; Chen, L.; Xie, L. Prediction of synergistic anti-cancer drug combinations based on the drug target network and drug-induced gene expression profiles. *Artif. Intell. Med.* 2017, 83, 35–43. https://doi.org/10.1016/j.artmed.2017.05.008.

45. Choudhury, C.; Murugan, N.A.; Priyakumar, U.D. Structure-based drug repurposing: Traditional and advanced AI/ML-aided methods. *Drug Discov. Today* 2022, 27, 1847–1861. https://doi.org/10.1016/j.drudis.2022.03.006.

46. Moll, S.; Desmoulière, A.; Moeller, M.J.; Pache, J.-C.; Badi, L.; Arcadu, F.; Richter, H.; Satz, A.; Uhles, S.; Cavalli, A.; et al. DDR1 role in fibrosis and its pharmacological targeting. *Biochim. Et Biophys. Acta (BBA)-Mol. Cell Res.* 2019, 1866, 118474. https://doi.org/10.1016/j.bbamcr.2019.04.004.

47. Ren, F.; Ding, X.; Zheng, M.; Korzinkin, M.; Cai, X.; Zhu, W.; Mantsyzov, A.; Aliper, A.; Aladinskiy, V.; Cao, Z.; et al. AlphaFold accelerates artificial intelligence powered drug discovery: Efficient discovery of a novel CDK20 small molecule inhibitor. *Chem. Sci.* 2023, 14, 1443–1452. https://doi.org/10.1039/d2sc05709c.

48. Deloitte-Intelligent Drug Discovery. (2023). Deloitte. Available online: https://www2.deloitte.com/content/dam/Deloitte/my/Documents/risk/my-risk-sdg3-intelligent-drug-discovery.pdf (accessed on 8 March 2023).

49. Dokholyan, N.V. Experimentally-driven protein structure modeling. *J. Proteom.* 2020, 220, 103777. https://doi.org/10.1016/j.jprot.2020.103777.

50. Greenfield, N.J. Using circular dichroism spectra to estimate protein secondary structure. *Nat. Protoc.* 2006, 1, 2876–2890. https://doi.org/10.1038/nprot.2006.202.

51. Bank, R.P.D. (2023). PDB Statistics: Protein-Only Structures Released Per Year. Available online: https://www.rcsb.org/stats/growth/growth-protein (accessed on 30 March 2023).

52. Mirdita, M.; Driesch, L.V.D.; Galiez, C.; Martin, M.-J.; Söding, J.; Steinegger, M. Uniclust databases of clustered and deeply annotated protein sequences and alignments. *Nucleic Acids Res.* 2017, 45, D170–D176. https://doi.org/10.1093/nar/gkw1081.

53. BFD. (n.d.). Available online: https://bfd.mmseqs.com/ (accessed on 30 March 2023).

54. Mitchell, A.L.; Scheremetjew, M.; Denise, H.; Potter, S.; Tarkowska, A.; Qureshi, M.; Salazar, G.A.; Pesseat, S.; Boland, M.A.; Hunter, F.; et al. EBI Metagenomics in 2017: Enriching the analysis of microbial communities, from sequence reads to assemblies. *Nucleic Acids Res.* 2018, 46, D726–D735. https://doi.org/10.1093/nar/gkx967.

55. Jumper, J.; Evans, R.; Pritzel, A.; Green, T.; Figurnov, M.; Ronneberger, O.; Tunyasuvunakool, K.; Bates, R.; Žídek, A.; Potapenko, A.; et al. Highly accurate protein structure prediction with AlphaFold. *Nature* 2021, 596, 583–589. https://doi.org/10.1038/s41586-021-03819-2.

56. Yang, J.; Anishchenko, I.; Park, H.; Peng, Z.; Ovchinnikov, S.; Baker, D. Improved protein structure prediction using predicted interresidue orientations. *Proc. Natl. Acad. Sci. USA* 2020, 117, 1496–1503. https://doi.org/10.1073/pnas.1914677117.

57. Du, Z.; Su, H.; Wang, W.; Ye, L.; Wei, H.; Peng, Z.; Anishchenko, I.; Baker, D.; Yang, J. The trRosetta server for fast and accurate protein structure prediction. *Nat. Protoc.* 2021, 16, 5634–5651. https://doi.org/10.1038/s41596-021-00628-9.

58. Kim, D.E.; Chivian, D.; Baker, D. Protein structure prediction and analysis using the Robetta server. *Nucleic Acids Res.* 2004, 32, W526–W531. https://doi.org/10.1093/nar/gkh468.

59. Baek, M.; DiMaio, F.; Anishchenko, I.; Dauparas, J.; Ovchinnikov, S.; Lee, G.R.; Wang, J.; Cong, Q.; Kinch, L.N.; Schaeffer, R.D.; et al. Accurate prediction of protein structures and interactions using a three-track neural network. *Science* 2021, 373, 871–876. https://doi.org/10.1126/science.abj8754.

60. Lin, Z.; Akin, H.; Rao, R.; Hie, B.; Zhu, Z.; Lu, W.; Smetanin, N.; Verkuil, R.; Kabeli, O.; Shmueli, Y.; et al. Language models of protein sequences at the scale of evolution enable accurate structure prediction. bioRxiv 2022. https://doi.org/10.1101/2022.07.20.500902.

61. Wu, R.; Ding, F.; Wang, R.; Shen, R.; Zhang, X.; Luo, S.; Su, C.; Wu, Z.; Xie, Q.; Berger, B.; et al. High-resolution de novo structure prediction from primary sequence. bioRxiv 2022. https://doi.org/10.1101/2022.07.21.500999.

62. AlphaFold Protein Structure Database. (2021). Available online: https://alphafold.ebi.ac.uk/ (accessed on 23 March 2023).

63. Roy, A.; Kucukural, A.; Zhang, Y. I-TASSER: A unified platform for automated protein structure and function prediction. *Nat. Protoc.* 2010, 5, 725–738. https://doi.org/10.1038/nprot.2010.5.

64. Yang, J.; Yan, R.; Roy, A.; Xu, D.; Poisson, J.; Zhang, Y. The I-TASSER Suite: Protein structure and function prediction. *Nat. Methods* 2015, 12, 7–8. https://doi.org/10.1038/nmeth.3213.

65. Waterhouse, A.; Bertoni, M.; Bienert, S.; Studer, G.; Tauriello, G.; Gumienny, R.; Heer, F.T.; De Beer, T.A.P.; Rempfer, C.; Bordoli, L.; et al. SWISS-MODEL: Homology modelling of protein structures and complexes. *Nucleic Acids Res.* 2018, 46, W296–W303. https://doi.org/10.1093/nar/gky427.

66. Fiser, A.; Šali, A. Modeller: Generation and refinement of homology-based protein structure models. *Methods Enzymol.* 2003, 374, 461–491. https://doi.org/10.1016/s0076-6879(03)74020-8.

67. Deng, H.; Jia, Y.; Zhang, Y. Protein structure prediction. *Int. J. Mod. Phys. B* 2018, 32(18), 1840009. https://doi.org/10.1142/s021797921840009x.

68. Segler, M.H.S.; Preuss, M.; Waller, M.P. Planning chemical syntheses with deep neural networks and symbolic AI. *Nature* 2018, 555, 604–610. https://doi.org/10.1038/nature25978.

69. Mak, K.-K.; Pichika, M.R. Artificial intelligence in drug development: Present status and future prospects. *Drug Discov. Today* 2019, 24, 773–780. https://doi.org/10.1016/j.drudis.2018.11.014.

70. Kosugi, T.; Ohue, M. Solubility-aware protein binding peptide design using AlphaFold. *Biomedicines* 2022, 10, 1626. https://doi.org/10.3390/biomedicines10071626.

71. Wong, F.; Krishnan, A.; Zheng, E.J.; Stärk, H.; Manson, A.L.; Earl, A.M.; Jaakkola, T.; Collins, J.J. Benchmarking AlphaFold-enabled molecular docking predictions for antibiotic discovery. *Mol. Syst. Biol.* 2022, 18, e11081. https://doi.org/10.15252/msb.202211081.

72. Available online: https://pandaomics.com/access (accessed on 23 March 2023).
73. Matsuzaka, Y.; Yashiro, R. Applications of deep learning for drug discovery systems with BigData. *BioMedinformatics* 2022, 2, 603–624. https://doi.org/10.3390/biomedinformatics2040039.
74. Wallach, I.; Dzamba, M.; Heifets, A. AtomNet: A deep convolutional neural network for bioactivity prediction in structure-based drug discovery. arXiv 2015. https://doi.org/10.48550/arXiv.1510.02855.
75. Öztürk, H.; Özgür, A.; Ozkirimli, E. DeepDTA: Deep drug-target binding affinity prediction. *Bioinformatics* 2018, 34, i821–i829. https://doi.org/10.1093/bioinformatics/bty593.
76. Ferreira, L.; Borba, J.; Moreira-Filho, J.; Rimoldi, A.; Andrade, C.; Costa, F. QSAR-based virtual screening of natural products database for identification of potent antimalarial hits. *Biomolecules* 2021, 11, 459. https://doi.org/10.3390/biom11030459.
77. Kanehisa, M.; Goto, S.; Kawashima, S.; Nakaya, A. The KEGG databases at GenomeNet. *Nucleic Acids Res.* 2002, 30, 42–46. https://doi.org/10.1093/nar/30.1.42.
78. Yao, Z.-J.; Dong, J.; Che, Y.-J.; Zhu, M.-F.; Wen, M.; Wang, N.-N.; Wang, S.; Lu, A.-P.; Cao, D.-S. TargetNet: A web service for predicting potential drug-target interaction profiling via multi-target SAR models. *J. Comput. Mol. Des.* 2016, 30, 413–424. https://doi.org/10.1007/s10822-016-9915-2.
79. Gentile, F.; Yaacoub, J.C.; Gleave, J.; Fernandez, M.; Ton, A.-T.; Ban, F.; Stern, A.; Cherkasov, A. Artificial intelligence-enabled virtual screening of ultra-large chemical libraries with deep docking. *Nat. Protoc.* 2022, 17, 672–697. https://doi.org/10.1038/s41596-021-00659-2.
80. Yang, C.; Chen, E.A.; Zhang, Y. Protein-ligand docking in the machine-learning era. *Molecules* 2022, 27, 4568. https://doi.org/10.3390/molecules27144568.
81. de Ruyck, J.; Brysbaert, G.; Blossey, R.; Lensink, M. Molecular docking as a popular tool in drug design, an in silico travel. *Adv. Appl. Bioinform. Chem.* 2016, 9, 1–11. https://doi.org/10.2147/AABC.S105289.
82. Trott, O.; Olson, A.J. AutoDock Vina: Improving the speed and accuracy of docking with a new scoring function, efficient optimization, and multithreading. *J. Comput. Chem.* 2010, 31, 455–461. https://doi.org/10.1002/jcc.21334.
83. Eberhardt, J.; Santos-Martins, D.; Tillack, A.F.; Forli, S. AutoDock Vina 1.2. 0: New docking methods, expanded force field, and python bindings. *J. Chem. Inf. Model.* 2021, 61, 3891–3898.
84. Venkatachalam, C.; Jiang, X.; Oldfield, T.; Waldman, M. LigandFit: A novel method for the shape-directed rapid docking of ligands to protein active sites. *J. Mol. Graph. Model.* 2003, 21, 289–307. https://doi.org/10.1016/s1093-3263(02)00164-x.
85. Allen, W.J.; Balius, T.E.; Mukherjee, S.; Brozell, S.R.; Moustakas, D.T.; Lang, P.T.; Case, D.A.; Kuntz, I.D.; Rizzo, R.C. DOCK 6: Impact of new features and current docking performance. *J. Comput. Chem.* 2015, 36, 1132–1156. https://doi.org/10.1002/jcc.23905.
86. Jones, G.; Willett, P.; Glen, R.C.; Leach, A.R.; Taylor, R. Development and validation of a genetic algorithm for flexible docking. *J. Mol. Biol.* 1997, 267, 727–748. https://doi.org/10.1006/jmbi.1996.0897.
87. Das, N.C.; Chakraborty, P.; Bayry, J.; Mukherjee, S. In silico analyses on the comparative potential of therapeutic human monoclonal antibodies against newly emerged SARS-CoV-2 variants bearing mutant spike protein. *Front. Immunol.* 2022, 12, 782506. https://doi.org/10.3389/fimmu.2021.782506.

88. Ramos, J.; Muthukumaran, J.; Freire, F.; Paquete-Ferreira, J.; Otrelo-Cardoso, A.R.; Svergun, D.; Panjkovich, A.; Santos-Silva, T. Shedding light on the interaction of human anti-apoptotic Bcl-2 protein with ligands through biophysical and in silico studies. *Int. J. Mol. Sci.* 2019, 20, 860. https://doi.org/10.3390/ijms20040860.

89. Neves, M.A.C.; Totrov, M.; Abagyan, R. Docking and scoring with ICM: The benchmarking results and strategies for improvement. *J. Comput. Mol. Des.* 2012, 26, 675–686. https://doi.org/10.1007/s10822-012-9547-0.

90. Friesner, R.A., Banks, J.L.; Murphy, R.B.; Halgren, T.A.; Klicic, J.J.; Mainz, D.T.; Repasky, M.P.; Knoll, E.H.; Shelley, M.; Perry, J.K.; et al., Glide: A new approach for rapid, accurate docking and scoring. 1. Method and assessment of docking accuracy. *J. Med. Chem.* 2004, 47, 1739–1749. https://doi.org/10.1021/jm0306430.

91. Bao, J.; He, X.; Zhang, J.Z.H. DeepBSP-A machine learning method for accurate prediction of protein-ligand docking structures. *J. Chem. Inf. Model.* 2021, 61, 2231–2240. https://doi.org/10.1021/acs.jcim.1c00334.

92. Yadav, P.; Mollaei, P.; Cao, Z.; Wang, Y.; Farimani, A.B. Prediction of GPCR activity using machine learning. *Comput. Struct. Biotechnol. J.* 2022, 20, 2564–2573. https://doi.org/10.1016/j.csbj.2022.05.016.

93. Vemula, D.; Jayasurya, P.; Sushmitha, V.; Kumar, Y.N.; Bhandari, V. CADD, AI and ML in drug discovery: A comprehensive review. *Eur. J. Pharm. Sci.* 2023, 181, 106324. https://doi.org/10.1016/j.ejps.2022.106324.

94. Guedes, I.A.; Pereira, F.S.S.; Dardenne, L.E. Empirical scoring functions for structure-based virtual screening: Applications, critical aspects, and challenges. *Front Pharmacol.* 2018, 9, 1089. https://doi.org/10.3389/fphar.2018.01089.

95. Pantsar, T.; Poso, A. Binding affinity via docking: Fact and fiction. *Molecules* 2018, 23, 1899. https://doi.org/10.3390/molecules23081899.

96. Böhm, H.-J. The development of a simple empirical scoring function to estimate the binding constant for a protein-ligand complex of known three-dimensional structure. *J. Comput. Mol. Des.* 1994, 8, 243–256. https://doi.org/10.1007/bf00126743.

97. Li, H.; Leung, K.-S.; Wong, M.-H.; Ballester, P.J. Low-quality structural and interaction data improves binding affinity prediction via random forest. *Molecules* 2015, 20, 10947–10962. https://doi.org/10.3390/molecules200610947.

98. de Magalhães, C.S.; Almeida, D.M.; Barbosa, H.J.C.; Dardenne, L.E. A dynamic niching genetic algorithm strategy for docking highly flexible ligands. *Inf. Sci.* 2014, 289, 206–224. https://doi.org/10.1016/j.ins.2014.08.002.

99. Debroise, T.; Shakhnovich, E.I.; Chéron, N. A Hybrid knowledge-based and empirical scoring function for protein-Ligand interaction: SMoG2016. *J. Chem. Inf. Model.* 2017, 57, 584–593. https://doi.org/10.1021/acs.jcim.6b00610.

100. Baek, M.; Shin, W.-H.; Chung, H.W.; Seok, C. GalaxyDock BP2 score: A hybrid scoring function for accurate protein-ligand docking. *J. Comput. Mol. Des.* 2017, 31, 653–666. https://doi.org/10.1007/s10822-017-0030-9.

101. Guedes, I.A.; Barreto, A.M.S.; Marinho, D.; Krempser, E.; Kuenemann, M.A.; Sperandio, O.; Dardenne, L.E.; Miteva, M.A. New machine learning and physics-based scoring functions for drug discovery. *Sci. Rep.* 2021, 11, 3198. https://doi.org/10.1038/s41598-021-82410-1.

102. McNutt, A.T.; Francoeur, P.; Aggarwal, R.; Masuda, T.; Meli, R.; Ragoza, M.; Sunseri, J.; Koes, D.R. GNINA 1.0: Molecular docking with deep learning. *J. Cheminform.* 2021, 13, 43. https://doi.org/10.1186/s13321-021-00522-2.

103. Lamberti, M.J. A study on the application and use of artificial intelligence to support drug development. *Clin. Ther.* 2019, 41, 1414–1426.

104. Choi, S.; Park, H.; Jung, S.; Kim, E.-K.; Cho, M.-L.; Min, J.-K.; Moon, S.-J.; Lee, S.-M.; Cho, J.-H.; Lee, D.-H.; et al. Therapeutic effect of exogenous truncated IK protein in inflammatory arthritis. *Int. J. Mol. Sci.* 2017, 18, 1976. https://doi.org/10.3390/ijms18091976.

105. Rigi, G.; Kardar, G.; Hajizade, A.; Zamani, J.; Ahmadian, G. The effects of a truncated form of Staphylococcus aureus protein A (SpA) on the expression of cytokines of autoimmune patients and healthy individuals. *Europe PMC* 2022. (not peer-reviewed). https://doi.org/10.21203/rs.3.rs-1635617/v1.

106. Xu, J.; Lloyd, D.J.; Hale, C.; Stanislaus, S.; Chen, M.; Sivits, G.; Vonderfecht, S.; Hecht, R.; Li, Y.-S.; Lindberg, R.A.; et al. Fibroblast growth factor 21 reverses hepatic steatosis, increases energy expenditure, and improves insulin sensitivity in diet-induced obese mice. *Diabetes* 2009, 58, 250–259. https://doi.org/10.2337/db08-0392.

107. Véniant, M.M.; Komorowski, R.; Chen, P.; Stanislaus, S.; Winters, K.; Hager, T.; Zhou, L.; Wada, R.; Hecht, R.; Xu, J. Long-acting FGF21 has enhanced efficacy in diet-induced obese mice and in obese rhesus monkeys. *Endocrinology* 2012, 153, 4192–4203. https://doi.org/10.1210/en.2012-1211.

108. Charych, D.H.; Hoch, U.; Langowski, J.L.; Lee, S.R.; Addepalli, M.K.; Kirk, P.B.; Sheng, D.; Liu, X.; Sims, P.W.; van der Veen, L.A.; et al. NKTR-214, an engineered cytokine with biased IL2 receptor binding, increased tumor exposure, and marked efficacy in mouse tumor models. *Clin. Cancer Res.* 2016, 22, 680–690. https://doi.org/10.1158/1078-0432.ccr-15-1631.

109. Peters, C.; Brown, S. Antibody-drug conjugates as novel anti-cancer chemotherapeutics. *Biosci. Rep.* 2015, 35, e00225. Available online: https://pubmed.ncbi.nlm.nih.gov/26182432/ (accessed on 23 March 2023).

110. Khongorzul, P.; Ling, C.J.; Khan, F.U.; Ihsan, A.U.; Zhang, J. Antibody-drug conjugates: A comprehensive review. *Mol. Cancer Res.* 2020, 18, 3–19. https://doi.org/10.1158/1541-7786.mcr-19-0582.

111. Fu, Z.; Li, S.; Han, S.; Shi, C.; Zhang, Y. Antibody drug conjugate: The "biological missile" for targeted cancer therapy. *Signal Transduct. Target. Ther.* 2022, 7, 1–25. https://doi.org/10.1038/s41392-022-00947-7.

112. Available online: https://www.bio-itworld.com/pressreleases/2022/11/28/fda-approved-adc-drugs-list-up-to-2022 (accessed on 23 March 2023).

113. McPherson, M.J.; Hobson, A.D. Pushing the envelope: Advancement of ADCs outside of oncology. In *Antibody-Drug Conjugates*, Tumey, L., Ed.; Humana: New York, 2020, vol. 2078, pp. 23–36. https://doi.org/10.1007/978-1-4939-9929-3_2.

114. Alley, S.C.; Okeley, N.M.; Senter, P.D. Antibody-drug conjugates: Targeted drug delivery for cancer. *Curr. Opin. Chem. Biol.* 2010, 14, 529–537.

115. Beck, A.; Haeuw, J.-F.; Wurch, T.; Goetsch, L.; Bailly, C.; Corvaïa, N. The next generation of antibody-drug conjugates comes of age. *Discov. Med.* 2010, 10, 329–359.

116. Ritter, A. Antibody-drug conjugates: Looking ahead to an emerging class of biotherapeutic. *Pharm. Tech.*.2012, 36, 42–47.

117. Junttila, T.T.; Li, G.; Parson, K.; Phillips, G.L.; Sliwkowski, M.X. Trastuzumab-DM1 (T-DM1) retains all the mechanisms of action of trastuzumab and efficiently inhibits growth of lapatinib-insensitive breast cancer. *Breast Cancer Res. Treat.* 2011, 128, 347–356.

118. Schmidt, M.M.; Wittrup, K.D. A modeling analysis of the effects of molecular size and binding affinity on tumor targeting. *Mol. Cancer Ther.* 2009, 8, 2861–2871.

119. Francisco, J.A.; Cerveny, C.G.; Meyer, D.L.; Mixan, B.J.; Klussman, K.; Chace, D.F.; Rejniak, S.X.; Gordon, K.A.; DeBlanc, R.; Toki, B.E.; et al. cAC10-vcMMAE, an anti-CD30-monomethyl auristatin E conjugate with potent and selective antitumor activity. *Blood* 2003, 102, 1458–1465. https://doi.org/10.1182/blood-2003-01-0039.

120. Kovtun, Y.V.; Goldmacher, V.S. Cell killing by antibody-drug conjugates. *Cancer Lett.* 2007, 255, 232–240. https://doi.org/10.1016/j.canlet.2007.04.010.

121. Baah, S.; Laws, M.; Rahman, K. Antibody-drug conjugates-a tutorial review. *Molecules* 2021, 26, 2943. https://doi.org/10.3390/molecules26102943.

122. Hebbrecht, T.; Liu, J.; Zwaenepoel, O.; Boddin, G.; Van Leene, C.; Decoene, K.; Madder, A.; Braeckmans, K.; Gettemans, J. Nanobody click chemistry for convenient site-specific fluorescent labelling, single step immunocytochemistry and delivery into living cells by photoporation and live cell imaging. *New Biotechnol.* 2020, 59, 33–43. https://doi.org/10.1016/j.nbt.2020.05.004.

123. Jaffray, D.A. Image-guided radiotherapy: From current concept to future perspectives. *Nat. Rev. Clin. Oncol.* 2012, 9, 688–699.

124. Nasr, D.; Kumar, P.A.; Zerdan, M.B.; Ghelani, G.; Dutta, D.; Graziano, S.; Lim, S.H. Radioimmunoconjugates in the age of modern immuno-oncology. *Life Sci.* 2022, 310, 121126. https://doi.org/10.1016/j.lfs.2022.121126.

125. Pouget, J.P.; Constanzo, J. Revisiting the radiobiology of targeted alpha therapy. *Front. Med.* 2018, 8, 692436.

126. Grillo-López, A.J. Zevalin: The first radioimmunotherapy approved for the treatment of lymphoma. *Expert. Rev. Anticancer Ther.* 2002, 2, 485–493.

127. Zaheer, J.; Kim, H.; Lee, Y.-J.; Kim, J.S.; Lim, S.M. Combination radioimmunotherapy strategies for solid tumors. *Int. J. Mol. Sci.* 2019, 20 (22): 5579. https://doi.org/10.3390/ijms20225579.

128. Miranda, A.C.C.; Santos, S.N.D.; Fuscaldi, L.L.; Balieiro, L.M.; Bellini, M.H.; Guimarães, M.I.C.C.; de Araújo, E.B. Radioimmunotheranostic pair based on the anti-HER2 monoclonal antibody: Influence of chelating agents and radionuclides on biological properties. *Pharmaceutics* 2021, 13, 971.

129. Chiu, K.; Racz, R.; Burkhart, K.; Florian, J.; Ford, K.; Garcia, M.I.; Geiger, R.M.; Howard, K.E.; Hyland, P.L.; Ismaiel, O.A.; et al. New science, drug regulation, and emergent public health issues: The work of FDA's division of applied regulatory science. *Front. Med.* 2023, 9, 03. https://doi.org/10.3389/fmed.2022.1109541.

130. U S Food and Drug Administration. Clinical Pharmacology Review for Application 214787Orig1S000 (Remdesivir). 2022. Available online: https://www.accessdata.fda.gov/drugsatfda_docs/nda/2020/214787Orig1s000ClinpharmR.pdf (accessed on 23 March 2023).

131. FDA. Available online: https://www.fda.gov/about-fda/center-drug-evaluation-and-research-cder/division-applied-regulatory-science (accessed on 23 March 2023).

132. Schotland, P.; Racz, R.; Jackson, D.B.; Soldatos, T.G.; Levin, R.; Strauss, D.G.; Burkhart, K. Target adverse event profiles for predictive safety in the postmarket setting. *Clin. Pharmacol. Ther.* 2020, 109, 1232–1243. https://doi.org/10.1002/cpt.2074.

133. Yan, H.; Bhagwat, B.; Sanden, D.; Willingham, A.; Tan, A.; Knapton, A.D.; Weaver, J.L.; Howard, K.E. Evaluation of a TGN1412 analogue using in vitro assays and two immune humanized mouse models. *Toxicol. Appl. Pharmacol.* 2019, 372, 57–69. https://doi.org/10.1016/j.taap.2019.03.020.

134. Yan, H.; Semple, K.M.; Gonzaléz, C.M.; Howard, K.E. Bone marrow-liver-thymus (BLT) immune humanized mice as a model to predict cytokine release syndrome. *Transl. Res.* 2019, 210, 43–56. https://doi.org/10.1016/j.trsl.2019.04.007.

135. Weaver, J.L.; Zadrozny, L.M.; Gabrielson, K.; Semple, K.M.; Shea, K.I.; Howard, K.E. BLT-Immune humanized mice as a model for nivolumab-induced immune-mediated adverse events: Comparison of the NOG and NOG-EXL strains. *Toxicol. Sci.* 2019, 169, 194–208. https://doi.org/10.1093/toxsci/kfz045.

136. Daluwatte, C.; Schotland, P.; Strauss, D.G.; Burkhart, K.K.; Racz, R. Predicting potential adverse events using safety data from marketed drugs. *BMC Bioinform.* 2020, 21, 163. https://doi.org/10.1186/s12859-020-3509-7.

137. Postoiaalliance, 2023. Available online: https://www.pistoiaalliance.org/ (accessed on 23 March 2023).
138. International Council for Harmonisation of Technical Requirements for Pharmaceuticals for Human Use [ICH]. Assessment and Control of DNA Reactive (mutagenic) Impurities in Pharmaceuticals to Limit Potential Carcinogenic Risk. M7(R1). Current Step 4 Version. 2017. Available online: https://database.ich. org/sites/default/files/M7_R1_ Guideline.pdf (accessed on 23 March 2023).
139. Convolutional Neural Networks. Available online: https://www.youtube.com/watch?v= bNb2fEVKeEo&t=6sExternal Link Disclaimer (accessed on 23 March 2023).
140. Particle Sentry AI: Quality Control in Drug Product Manufacturing. Available online: https://www.semitorr.com/specialties/particle-sentry-ai-quality-control-in-drug-prod- uct-manufacturing/ (accessed on 23 March 2023).
141. FDA Approved Drugs Available online: https://www.accessdata.fda.gov/scripts/cder/ daf/index.cfm (accessed on 23 March 2023).
142. FDA AccessData. Available online: https://www.ema.europa.eu/en/medicines/ what-we-publish-when/european-public-assessment-reports-background-context (accessed on 23 March 2023).
143. Niazi, S. A Modified 351(a) Licensing Pathway for Biosimilars Available online: https://www.centerforbiosimilars.com/view/opinion-a-modified-351-a-licensing-path- way-for-biosimilars (accessed on 23 March 2023).
144. Wang, Y.C.; Wang, Y.; Schrieber, S.J.; Earp, J.; Thway, T.M.; Huang, S.M.; Zineh, I.; Christl, L. Role of modeling and simulation in the development of novel and biosimilar therapeutic proteins. *J. Pharm. Sci.* 2019, 108, 73–77.
145. Wang, Y.; Huang, S.M. Commentary on fit-for-purpose models for regulatory applica- tions. *J. Pharm. Sci.* 2019, 108, 18–20. https://doi.org/10.1016/j.xphs.2018.09.009.
146. Zhu, P.; Hsu, C.-H.; Liao, J.; Xu, S.; Zhang, L.; Zhou, H. Trial design and statistical considerations on the assessment of pharmacodynamic similarity. *AAPS J.* 2019, 21, 47. https://doi.org/10.1208/s12248-019-0321-2.
147. Zhu, P.; Ji, P.; Wang, Y. Using Clinical PK/PD studies to support no clinically meaning- ful differences between a proposed biosimilar and the reference product. *AAPS J.* 2018, 20, 89. https://doi.org/10.1208/s12248-018-0246-1.
148. US Food and Drug Administration. FDA Guidance: Bioanalytical Method Validation. 2018. Available online: https://www.fda.gov/media/70858/ download (accessed on 1 April 2022).
149. Lim, S.H.; Kim, K.; Choi, C.-I. Pharmacogenomics of monoclonal antibodies for the treatment of rheumatoid arthritis. *J. Pers. Med.* 2022, 12, 1265. https://doi.org/10.3390/ jpm12081265.
150. Niazi, S. Volume of distribution as a function of time. *J. Pharm. Sci.* 1976, 65, 452–454. https://doi.org/10.1002/jps.2600650339. Available online: https://www.sciencedirect. com/science/article/abs/pii/S0022354915406495 (accessed on 23 March 2023).
151. Wesolowski, C.; Wesolowski, M.J.; Babyn, P.S.; Wanasundara, S.N. Time varying apparent volume of distribution and drug half-lives following intravenous bolus injec- tions. *PLoS ONE* 2016, 11, e0158798. https://doi.org/10.1371/journal.pone.0158798.
152. Gadkar, K.; Yadav, D.B.; Zuchero, J.Y.; Couch, J.A.; Kanodia, J.; Kenrick, M.K.; Atwal, J.K.; Dennis, M.S.; Prabhu, S.; Watts, R.J.; et al. Mathematical PKPD and safety model of bispecific TfR/BACE1 antibodies for the optimization of antibody uptake in brain. *Eur. J. Pharm. Biopharm.* 2016, 101, 53–61.
153. Wittrup, K.D.; Thurber, G.M.; Schmidt, M.M.; Rhoden, J.J. Practical theoretic guid- ance for the design of tumor-targeting agents. *Methods Enzymol.* 2012, 503, 255–268. https://doi.org/10.1016/b978-0-12-396962-0.00010-0.

154. Yeung, Y.A.; Leabman, M.K.; Marvin, J.S.; Qiu, J.; Adams, C.W.; Lien, S.; Starovasnik, M.A.; Lowman, H.B. Engineering human IgG1 affinity to human neonatal Fc receptor: Impact of affinity improvement on pharmacokinetics in primates. *J. Immunol.* 2009, 182, 7663–7671. https://doi.org/10.4049/jimmunol.0804182.

155. Deng, R.; Loyet, K.M.; Lien, S.; Iyer, S.; Deforge, L.E.; Theil, F.-P.; Lowman, H.B.; Fielder, P.J.; Prabhu, S. Pharmacokinetics of humanized monoclonal anti-tumor necrosis factor-α antibody and its neonatal Fc receptor variants in mice and cynomolgus monkeys. *Drug Metab. Dispos.* 2010, 38, 600–605. https://doi.org/10.1124/dmd.109.031310.

156. Robbie, G.J.; Criste, R.; Dall'Acqua, W.F.; Jensen, K.; Patel, N.K.; Losonsky, G.A.; Griffin, M.P. A Novel investigational Fc-modified humanized monoclonal antibody, motavizumab-YTE, has an extended half-life in healthy adults. *Antimicrob. Agents Chemother.* 2013, 57, 6147–6153. https://doi.org/10.1128/aac.01285-13.

157. Kamath, A.V. Translational pharmacokinetics and pharmacodynamics of monoclonal antibodies. *Drug Discov. Today Technol.* 2016, 21–22, 75–83. https://doi.org/10.1016/j.ddtec.2016.09.004.

158. Castelli, M.S.; McGonigle, P.; Hornby, P.J. The pharmacology and therapeutic applications of monoclonal antibodies. *Pharmacol. Res. Perspect.* 2019, 7, e00535. https://doi.org/10.1002/prp2.535.

159. Sweeney, G. Variability in the human drug response. *Thromb. Res.* 1983, 29, 3–15. https://doi.org/10.1016/0049-3848(83)90353-5.

160. Marchant, B. Pharmacokinetic factors influencing variability in human drug response. *Scand. J. Rheumatol.* 1981, 10, 5–14. https://doi.org/10.3109/03009748109095328.

161. Babin, V.; Taran, F.; Audisio, D. Late-stage carbon-14 labeling and isotope exchange: Emerging opportunities and future challenges. *JACS Au* 2022, 2, 1234–1251. https://doi.org/10.1021/jacsau.2c00030.

162. Holford, N.H.; Sheiner, L.B. Kinetics of pharmacologic response. *Pharmacol. Ther.* 1982, 16, 143–166. https://doi.org/10.1016/0163-7258(82)90051-1.

163. Keutzer, L.; You, H.; Farnoud, A.; Nyberg, J.; Wicha, S.G.; Maher-Edwards, G.; Vlasakakis, G.; Moghaddam, G.K.; Svensson, E.M.; Menden, M.P.; et al. Machine learning and pharmacometrics for prediction of pharmacokinetic data: Differences, similarities and challenges illustrated with rifampicin. *Pharmaceutics* 2022, 14, 1530. https://doi.org/10.3390/pharmaceutics14081530.

164. Cai, W.; Leil, T.; Gibiansky, L.; Krishna, M.; Zhang, H.; Gu, H.; Sun, H.; Throup, J.; Banerjee, S.; Girgis, I. Modeling and simulation of the pharmacokinetics and target engagement of an antagonist monoclonal antibody to interferon-γ-induced protein 10, BMS-986184, in healthy participants to guide therapeutic dosing. *Clin. Pharmacol. Drug Dev.* 2020, 9, 689–698. https://doi.org/10.1002/cpdd.784.

165. McClellan, J.E.; Conlon, H.D.; Bolt, M.W.; Kalfayan, V.; Palaparthy, R.; Rehman, M.I.; Kirchhoff, C.F. The 'totality-of-the-evidence' approach in the development of PF-06438179/GP1111, an infliximab biosimilar, and in support of its use in all indications of the reference product. *Ther. Adv. Gastroenterol.* 2019, 12. https://doi.org/10.1177/1756284819852535.

166. Ryding, J.; Stahl, M.; Ullmann, M. Demonstrating biosimilar and originator antidrug antibody binding comparability in antidrug antibody assays: A practical approach. *Bioanalysis* 2017, 9, 1395–1406. https://doi.org/10.4155/bio-2017-0111.

167. Wang, X.; An, Z.; Luo, W.; Xia, N.; Zhao, Q. Molecular and functional analysis of monoclonal antibodies in support of biologics development. *Protein Cell* 2018, 9, 74–85. https://doi.org/10.1007/s13238-017-0447-x.

168. Todoroki, K.; Yamada, T.; Mizuno, H.; Toyo'Oka, T. Current mass spectrometric tools for the bioanalyses of therapeutic monoclonal antibodies and antibody-drug conjugates. *Anal. Sci.* 2018, 34, 397–406. https://doi.org/10.2116/analsci.17r003.

169. Láng, J.A.; Balogh, Z.C.; Nyitrai, M.F.; Juhász, C.; Gilicze, A.K.B.; Iliás, A.; Zólyomi, Z.; Bodor, C.; Rábai, E. In vitro functional characterization of biosimilar therapeutic antibodies. *Drug Discov. Today Technol.* 2020, 37, 41–50. https://doi.org/10.1016/j.ddtec.2020.11.010.

170. Cymera, F.; Becka, H.; Rohde, A.; Reusch, D. Therapeutic monoclonal antibody N-glycosylation-Structure, function and therapeutic potential. *Biologicals* 2018, 52, 1–11.

171. Prior, S.; Hufton, S.E.; Fox, B.; Dougall, T.; Rigsby, P.; Bristow, A.; Participants of the study. International standards for monoclonal antibodies to support pre- and post-marketing product consistency: Evaluation of a candidate international standard for the bioactivities of rituximab. *MAbs* 2018, 10, 129–142. https://doi.org/10.1080/19420862.2017.1386824.

172. Hofmann, H.-P.; Kronthaler, U.; Fritsch, C.; Grau, R.; Müller, S.O.; Mayer, R.; Seidl, A.; Da Silva, A. Characterization and non-clinical assessment of the proposed etanercept biosimilar GP2015 with originator etanercept (Enbrel(r)). *Expert Opin. Biol. Ther.* 2016, 16, 1185–1195. https://doi.org/10.1080/14712598.2016.1217329.

173. FDA: Clinical Immunogenicity Considerations for Biosimilar and Interchangeable Insulin Products. Available online: https://www.fda.gov/regulatory-information/search-fda-guidance-documents/clinical-immunogenicity-considerations-biosimilar-and-interchangeable-insulin-products (accessed on 23 March 2023).

174. Zhou, S.-F.; Zhong, W.-Z. Drug design and discovery: Principles and applications. *Molecules* 2017, 22, 279. https://doi.org/10.3390/molecules22020279.

175. Michael Schlanker Publications. Available online: https://michaelschlander.com/publications-since-2020.html?file=files/downloads/publications/2018/Schlander-et-al-Cost-Drug-Development-2021-PharmacoEconomics.pdf&cid=5702#:~:text=Results%20Estimates%20of%20total%20average,%244.54%20billion%20(2019%20US%24) (accessed on 23 March 2023).

Index

Note: **Bold** page numbers refer to tables and *italic* page numbers refer to figures.

For Product Safety Concerns and Information please contact our EU
representative GPSR@taylorandfrancis.com
Taylor & Francis Verlag GmbH, Kaufingerstraße 24, 80331 München, Germany

www.ingramcontent.com/pod-product-compliance
Lightning Source LLC
Chambersburg PA
CBHW052013230326
41598CB00078B/3219

9 781032 519586